WOUND HEALING SECRETS

WOUND HEALING SECRETS

REVOLUTIONARY METHODS TO HEAL YOUR WOUND, SAVE YOUR LEG, AND RECLAIM YOUR LIFE!

JULIE HAMILTON, MD AND ROB HAMILTON, MD

Advantage®

Published by Advantage, Charleston, South Carolina.
Member of Advantage Media Group.

ADVANTAGE is a registered trademark and the Advantage colophon is a trademark of Advantage Media Group, Inc.

Printed in the United States of America.

ISBN: 978-1-59932-822-5
LCCN: 2017946903

Cover design by Katie Biondo and George Stevens.

This publication is designed to provide accurate and authoritative information in regard to the subject matter covered. It is sold with the understanding that the publisher is not engaged in rendering legal, accounting, or other professional services. If legal advice or other expert assistance is required, the services of a competent professional person should be sought.

Advantage Media Group is proud to be a part of the Tree Neutral® program. Tree Neutral offsets the number of trees consumed in the production and printing of this book by taking proactive steps such as planting trees in direct proportion to the number of trees used to print books. To learn more about Tree Neutral, please visit **www.treeneutral.com.**

Advantage Media Group is a publisher of business, self-improvement, and professional development books. We help entrepreneurs, business leaders, and professionals share their Stories, Passion, and Knowledge to help others Learn & Grow. Do you have a manuscript or book idea that you would like us to consider for publishing? Please visit **advantagefamily.com** or call **1.866.775.1696.**

Dedicated to our three sons: Max, Quinn and Jack.

To those with wounds, may you find healing in these pages.

With gratitude to Dr. Jack Kruse and Dr. Edward and Ly Kondrot.

TABLE OF CONTENTS

FOREWORD ix

INTRODUCTION 1

CHAPTER 1 13
Don't Let Them Take Your Leg!

CHAPTER 2 23
The Diabetes Apocalypse

CHAPTER 3 37
With Diabetes, Even a Scratch Can Kill

CHAPTER 4 43
Failures of the Medical System

CHAPTER 5 49
Wound Centers Offer Help

CHAPTER 6 57
Heal Yourself, Heal Your Wound

CHAPTER 7 67
Timing is Everything: An Introduction to Circadian Biology

CHAPTER 8 83
Eat Better to Heal Better

CHAPTER 9 95
Optimize Your Hormones

CHAPTER 10 . . . . **117**
Supplement Yourself

CHAPTER 11 . . . . **131**
Unravel the Mystery of Wound Healing

CHAPTER 12 . . . . **141**
Strategies to Help You Heal

CHAPTER 13 . . . . **151**
Heal with Steel

CHAPTER 14 . . . . **159**
Dressings: Pour Some Honey on That

CHAPTER 15 . . . . **171**
Even More Hope for Healing

CHAPTER 16 . . . . **179**
Infected or Not?

CHAPTER 17 . . . . **187**
Oxygen Heals

CHAPTER 18 . . . . **199**
Advanced and Alternative Therapies

CHAPTER 19 . . . . **213**
Regenerative Medicine: Your Body's Own Repair Kit

CHAPTER 20 . . . . **229**
Introducing the Quantlet

CHAPTER 21 . . . . **237**
Next Steps: Your Pathway to Healing

FOREWORD

Nature's health laws are quite simple. The road to health and happiness is not the labyrinthine maze described by our medical mystagogues. In pursuing their dietetic cedes, we learned in our training one becomes fairly bewildered by a mass of incongruous precepts and prescriptions. Why is that? I believe it is because these ideas are divorced from other aspects of nature like the power of sunlight. In medicine, we often are forced to make laborious compromises between old and new theories, arbitrary rules, and illogical exceptions, anti-natural restrictions, and anti-natural remedies. Their view of the constitution of man suggests the King of Aragon's remark about the cycles and epicycles of the Ptolemaic system: "It strikes me the Creator might have arranged this business in a simpler way."

With respect to wound healing in our modern world, there are a lot of modern ideas that use new technologies, but the best medicine always takes the thermodynamic givens that nature gives our cells as the base rate for the best success. Many times you'll hear physicians give you data and numbers on therapies and treatments. Most of those numbers are based upon probabilities. The mathematics that control this decision process is called Bayesian mathematics.

If you are reading this book you likely are trying to heal a tissue or avoid getting a wound. If you are wise, you will use your wounds and turn them into wisdom. Nature provides us with the base rate knowledge for wound healing. Most people with non-healing wounds have lost sight of that connection with nature, and they have to rely on their physicians and healthcare team to help rebuild and regenerate their bodies. Inside this book, between many of the words is the wisdom to enlighten the physician inside of your mind. This "doctor" can augment the information Doctors Julie and Rob Hamilton are trying to give you on the pages. To help them help yourself, you'd be wise to begin to use those things buried inside of you. Sometimes it is the simple things that help us the most. Taking your shoes off, sitting in the sunlight, and becoming reacquainted with your nature might be just what the doctor ordered!

Sunlight provides plants and animals with a constant source of energy. We often forget the natural healing built into the light of the sun. Every time we eat we should remind ourselves that the sun's light creates every last foodstuff on this planet. In a leaf, the reaction center acts as a solar battery that generates a small electrical potential from sunlight. That little spark of electricity is what makes food by photosynthesis.

Way back in the 1970s, Dr. Robert O. Becker, MD, a pioneering surgeon at Syracuse Medical University, made a startling discovery after he started using electrically generated silver ions to heal severe cases of osteomyelitis, a bone infection that can open up large wounds in a patient's flesh. He found that the use of silver ions amplified a small DC electric current from a simple nine-volt battery so that a difficult bone wound might heal. He got the idea from nature and how plants heal after an insect bites into a leaf to eat it.

By generating silver ions directly into open infected wounds through the use of a small, battery-operated colloidal silver generator operating at 0.9 volts, he found that not only did the silver effectively kill the infectious micro-organisms responsible for the disease, but it also triggered amazing and quite unexpected regrowth of human tissue and bone at the site of the infection.

In other words, far from damaging human cells, Becker discovered that silver caused astonishing cellular repair, resulting in dramatic healing of damaged tissues. Becker became the first researcher to discover that electrically generated silver ions have the power to not only kill pathogens and heal infections but also to stimulate tissue and bone regrowth. I learned about this work when I was studying to become a neurosurgeon in the early 1990s. I was astonished at his work. I was more astonished that we were not taking more advantage of the power of light to make electric currents in our patients with poor wound healing. That was the first time I learned about the power of nature built into our species by Mother Nature.

I wanted to share this story with you because you can help your doctors by tapping that unused potential inside of your tissues with the guidance of your physicians. There is a lot of good data in the subsequent pages designed to help you overcome poor tissue regeneration, but you can do a lot more to make it successful. Most of what you need to consider is not that hard to do. Who would have thought a small nine-volt battery and some silver could mimic what sunlight is capable of!

Health is merely the slowest form of death we create. Wound healing is how we delay illness and dying.

What is my take-home message before you begin to read this book? Sunrises and sunsets are clinics dispensing free care for wounds. Physics drives our biology and opens the door to the compound pharmacy in our pituitary. Our pituitary provides our tissues with a compound pharmacy of solutions that can heal the most stubborn wounds. Every sunset is a reset, a chance to regenerate something inside of you to help you. Every sunrise collapses a new waveform, a new possibility inside that you might not have fully realized yet. When you live in an optimized environment with ideal optics, most ailments can be cured; time can be slowed using frequencies of light while surgery can be done by you on your surroundings to guarantee repair. Putting Windex on your glass eye of beliefs is brain surgery without a scalpel that can bring you health once again.

Humans enter this world and awaken to a simple truth: First we must find our voice to flourish. Everyone is built to look forward, toward their specific future. In the beginning, we hear only our own noises as infants. Infants are magnificent creatures who remain affixed to the present moment. With time, they learn to listen to the echoes of past deeds, done by their own actions, returning their focus and attention to the past. This is very short-sighted because life causes every infant to go very far from where they began. It's unfathomable that this is what some of us are still focusing upon right now. That optic hinders our ability to heal. This is why famous songs are written about people who still cannot find what they are looking for. Focusing on the rearview mirror of your life only invites grief to your life. Grief breeds stress and stress stops healing.

Grief loves a hollow space in our mind; all it wants to do is to hear its own echo. Grief throws its words into the silence, and it always seems to find its echo somewhere where that silence opens hidden lexicons to ruin our future ability to heal. For people like this, their wounds become a canyon whose walls reverberate with a symphony of echoing words from earthly acts and choices they cannot escape. Our echoes should trail off almost forever on the horizon in our mind when we are healing because we must choose to focus toward the windshield of our life. These echoes cause a season of mistrust about the future to fog our mindset. Mistrust of our future makes it hard to give up past beliefs that our scars remind us of. For some, the echoes of the wound or the scar become more substantial than the acts that created them were themselves, but many never learn that lesson because they remain focused in the past and not the present. Stress of any kind will hinder your recovery.

Master the ego; embrace your fears, your anxieties, and your darkest thoughts; and channel them into the requisite energy and emotional intensity of nature to help your doctors heal you. Strong words resonate, but echoes are always more noisy than the source, and they should lead us to change to get the regeneration we seek.

The only ones who can help them are themselves. Are you ready yet? Are you ready to read a book that can alter the trajectory of your present wound or will you continue to listen to echoes of the origin of that wound?

You don't build a business in my world. You build people, and this book in your hands is fully capable of helping you achieve that goal. Maybe, if the authors are lucky, some of you reading this book might begin to help them build a natural healing workshop for mankind. We must get our mission correct when we are helping the ill, and the mission of this book is to help you help yourself today to do just that.

The conversations are always crazy deep between nature and humans with troubling wounds. Healers are trying to change the present reality that a wound creates for patients. Humans with poor healing wounds often feel broken. Humans are not broken, but the environment they have built is often hindering their healing below their perception level. We are created for uniqueness, and we are quantum beings now living in a synthetic world. That world has created many things that hinder our ability to heal. You'll learn, as you get wiser by reading this book, that some rules are made to be broken to regain what we've lost. Be bold enough to live life on your terms, and never, ever apologize for it. Sometimes *not following* the herd has its benefits in healing a difficult wound.

The story of Dr. Becker is a classic example of what I faced early on in my own training. It taught me to search for deeper answers when the textbooks were not helping my patients heal properly. Sometimes going back to nature and going against the grain and refusing to conform has some benefits in tough cases. Your doctor's advice, along with your intuition, can help your transition back to health from a nasty wound. Sometimes using uncommon methods built into nature are akin to taking the road less traveled instead of the well-beaten path. It might be the part of the prescription you are missing to heal that stubborn wound. Sometimes we need to laugh in the face of adversity and leap before we look when we get stumped in healthcare. Remaining positive and optimistic is as important with wound healing as any technique I have ever used as a surgeon.

Dr. Jack Kruse
New Orleans, Louisiana
January 2017
Author, *The Epi-Paleo Rx*
www.jackkruse.com

References and Recommended Reading

1. Robert O. Becker, "Effects of Electrically Generated Silver Ions on Human Cells and Wound Healing," *Journal of Electro- and Magnetobiology* 19, no. 1: 1–19 (2000).

INTRODUCTION

DO YOU HAVE A WOUND?

Are you one of the nearly seven million Americans—or uncounted millions worldwide—with a non-healing wound? Have you seen several different doctors, been given all manner of recommendations, and tried multiple treatments? Are you experiencing pain, isolation, fear, and frustration? We can help you.

No matter where your wound is—your foot, leg, abdomen, sacral area (lower back)—it is miserable. You may be too embarrassed to go out into public even if you keep it covered. Sometimes chronic wounds have a foul smell and drain pus or serous (watery) fluid that soaks through dressings. Some chronic wounds are painful, no matter whether dressed or exposed to air. You may develop allergic skin irritations from your drainage or the dressings. Chronic wounds increase inflammation within your body and may make every part of you hurt. They definitely age you more quickly.

Your wound and your overall health and vitality are inextricably intertwined; improving one absolutely improves the other, sometimes in startling and amazing ways. Healing *you* will heal your wound, and as your wound heals, so you will heal.

We are Doctors Julie and Rob Hamilton. We both trained in and practiced emergency medicine, but we have since followed our passions and our curiosity into other fields of medicine—wound care (Dr. Julie) and anti-aging and regenerative medicine (Dr. Rob). We have combined the latest techniques in advanced wound care and anti-aging/regenerative medicine. It is our passion to help you heal your wound, save your limb, improve your health, and reclaim your life.

Let us introduce ourselves so you understand our journey, experience, expertise, and cutting-edge ideas.

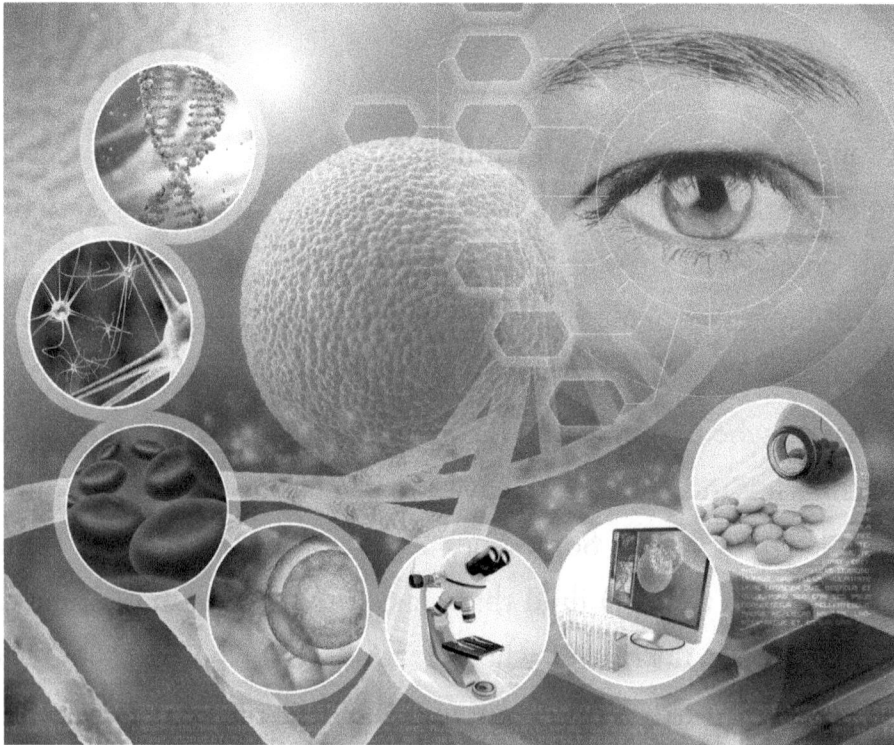

DR. JULIE'S STORY

While pursuing my MD degree at Stanford Medical School, several formative experiences piqued an interest in wound care. I helped organize a medical mission trip to Papua New Guinea. Our group traveled by dugout canoe to the remote Sepik River region, and I will never forget trying to help a sadly disfigured thirteen-year-old girl with yaws (a skin infection caused by the *Treponema pallidum* bacteria). As the flies swarmed about, I tried in vain to cover and protect all the ulcers on her arms, legs, and face. After running out of antibiotic ointment and gauze, I tried using banana leaves tied on with torn strips from my t-shirt. What she really needed was a three-day canoe trip to the nearest health clinic where she could receive shots of penicillin (an effective treatment). We recommended this to the village elders, but I never knew if they allowed her to go. A few weeks after I had cared for her weeping ulcers, I contracted yaws myself. Penicillin eradicated my infection and prevented me from developing similar wounds.

I also lived for a time on the Indonesian island of Sulawesi in an area endemic for typhoid fever. I collected blood samples to evaluate and test a new typhoid vaccine. At the health clinics, I treated a variety of tropical ulcers, skin infections, and wounds. There I learned and grew to respect some very effective, centuries-old, natural remedies.

When it came time to choose a specialty, emergency medicine seemed a natural fit because of my interests in travel and wilderness medicine. After completing residency training at both UC San Diego and Stanford, I practiced emergency medicine for the next ten years at a trauma center in Northern California.

Although not as glamorous as resuscitating patients, my ER training provided confidence and knowledge in treating critical wounds; they were cleaned, explored, packed, sutured, stapled, and dressed as needed. Some wounds warranted prophylactic antibiotics, tetanus boosters, or a trip to the OR with a surgeon.

Unfortunately, however, I had not received any training in the treatment of chronic wounds. I would "disinfect" the wounds with Betadine (I have since learned how caustic this is for healing tissues) and prescribe "wet-to-dry" dressings, triple antibiotic ointment, Silvadene cream, or Xeroform (a yellow, non-stick gauze). I usually prescribed antibiotics (because all chronic wounds "appeared" infected) and recommended follow-up. If the patient was very ill or had failed outpatient antibiotics, I would administer intravenous (IV) antibiotics and admit them to the hospital.

Most primary care doctors did not know what to do either when the wound remained non-healed at follow-up (other than prescribe more antibiotics). No doctors in our community had expertise in helping these patients heal, so many eventually returned to the emergency department. What a sad and frustrating cycle for the patient. I aspired to learn more and do better.

I traveled to Nix Medical Center (Texas) and Ohio State University for training in wound care as well as hyperbaric medicine (for the treatment of problem wounds). Dr. Rob and I were two of the original physicians to work at our local wound care center, which opened in 2008. I have enjoyed the multidisciplinary approach to healing the most challenging wounds. We treat every wound type, including those caused by diabetes, arterial and venous insufficiency, lymphedema, pressure, trauma, surgery, burns, autoimmune disease, malignancy, radiation, and a multitude of other problems. I have been the medical director since 2013. I work closely with the program director and staff to improve healing rates, and I frequently lecture to other doctors, nurses, and patients in our region.

I obtained board certification in undersea and hyperbaric medicine in 2012, because as of yet there is no widely agreed upon board certification for physicians in wound care medicine. As an Advanced Open Water SCUBA diver, I had always been interested in hyperbaric oxygen therapy (HBOT)—it is the primary treatment for "the bends," a condition that afflicts some divers (I almost needed it while diving the Great Barrier Reef during college). In reality, there are far more people benefitting from HBOT for wound healing than for any SCUBA diving related problems.

Although well versed in the best wound care practices of mainstream medicine, I have continued the quest to hone my craft and do better for my patients. Years of clinical experience have opened my eyes to the epidemic proportion of Americans suffering from chronic wounds and the failures of our medical system. We waste time and resources focused on the wound itself, instead of striving to understand the underlying cause. Many incredibly effective, advanced, alternative methods exist which we cannot put into practice at our hospital-based, insurance-billing, wound care center.

Although we have a highly performing center (as numbers go), sadly, some patients never heal or still end up with amputations despite the best care we deliver. We are limited by patient compliance, delayed referrals, bureaucratic pre-approval processes, and insurance company rules and limitations on breakthrough new therapies. Nothing is more frustrating than to be told that a patient's insurance will not cover a therapy that I know would be beneficial, and this is happening with increasing regularity.

My days in the wound clinic are very busy supervising HBOT; going from room to room to debride wounds; applying advanced dressings, tissue products, and grafts; and creating the mountain of documentation that insurance companies require to pay for the treatment. During those days, I have very limited time to explore, discuss, and explain all the underlying causes of wounds and how to correct them with my patients. I try hard, but I have even less time to discuss the importance of optimizing their health, hormones, nutrition, sleep, light environment, detoxification, gut-health, and mitochondrial health. Hours are needed, and I have only minutes.

The one thing that I have learned is that healing wounds quickly is critical to decreasing the risk of infection, hospitalization, and amputation. Accelerating the healing process also dramatically reduces costs.

The worldwide economic burden of diabetes is now estimated at around $1.3 trillion … and rising. Diabetic wounds contribute significantly to this cost. The medical profession should be more interested in preventing or reversing type 2 diabetes, not simply treating it. Prescribing insulin is not the answer. This book will teach lifestyle and dietary changes to help cure your disease.

We are writing this book to bring new knowledge to anyone interested in health and healing, which go hand in hand. We want to enable you to make educated and intelligent decisions about your healthcare options. Many people are beginning to see the failures of the pharmaceutical-driven, mainstream, and conventional medicine model whose costs are rising more rapidly than anyone can afford.

I treasure the relationships I develop with my patients. I have learned so much about the challenges and the misery that they face. They fear not only the isolation, embarrassment, odor, and pain associated with having chronic wounds; they also worry about the financial consequences. Many can no longer work or be productive. The costs of care, insurance co-pays, dressing supplies, and treatments add up quickly. Many feel guilty for being a burden to their loved ones. Some live in constant fear of an amputation. Others see their chronic wounds as a slow sign of dying. Their quality of life plummets.

My heart goes out to these people and the courageous course they steer through a medical system that is far from exceptional at taking care of their wounds, and even less so of their health and vitality.

Many people have given up hope, as they have been trying for years to heal. I love taking on this challenge, and we truly celebrate when their chronic wound transforms into an actively healing one. Seeing my patients avoid amputations and regain their lives and ability to function is truly a privilege, and I am thankful every day for this opportunity.

DR. ROB HAMILTON'S STORY

I have always been intensely curious and wanted to understand the smallest details of how the natural world works. My interest in the sciences was ignited by my father, a chemistry professor. I can remember him starting to teach me the details of organic chemistry and building molecular models with me as a child. Some of my first "tinker-toys" were actually his stick models of atoms and molecules.

I pursued a degree in electrical and computer engineering at the University of Colorado in Boulder. It was a rigorous and challenging course of study, but I relished the opportunity to understand every detail of how computers were built, from the electromagnetic theory, quantum physics, and semiconductor theory that depended on the physical chemistry (or was it the chemistry that depended on the physics?) to the logic design and higher-level programming. Little did I know how that background in semiconductor theory and quantum processes would come back to serve me well (haunt me?) as a physician.

After college, I decided to pursue medical school, wanting to learn more about how the human body worked. I was fascinated by every field of medicine and so chose emergency medicine as a specialty. It was a "jack of all trades and master of none" at a frenetic and sometimes terrifying pace, but I gained confidence in my skills and ability to take care of the worst acute injuries and illnesses.

For twenty years since medical school, I trained in and practiced emergency medicine. I have been involved at every level of the specialty, from bedside practice to the administration of a large physician group. I have developed expertise in dealing with the bureaucracy that doctors must deal with in order to provide patient care. I have taken care of nearly all types of injury, illness, and disease. I have been intimately involved in the crucible of emotions that occurs in the emergency department. I have been grateful to interact with many excellent physicians, nurses, paramedics, nurse practitioners, PAs, and other healthcare providers.

Over the years, as I have interfaced with nearly every medical specialty, I have developed an in-depth understanding of most of mainstream medicine. That is not to say I know all the details of each and every disease process or can do all the surgeries and procedures, nor can I prescribe every pharmaceutical for every condition. However, I do have a good sense for what is and what is not known and understood.

Unfortunately, this knowledge has left me with a sense of disquiet and an uneasy feeling. Despite all the amazing technological advances in medicine, despite the hundreds of thousands of medical research studies, and despite hundreds of modern pharmaceuticals and advanced surgical procedures and knowledge, from my ringside seat in the emergency department, the population of the United States is getting sicker faster than ever before.

For example, just a few short years ago when I was in residency, we were taught that type 2 diabetes was a disease of the elderly and that strokes and heart attacks were rare in people under the age of sixty. That is no longer the case in the day-to-day practice of medicine. Most doctors (especially ER doctors) know it is not uncommon to see patients in their twenties and thirties with diabetes, dyslipidemia, strokes, heart attacks, and neurological diseases like MS and early onset Alzheimer's disease that were thought to be diseases of much older people just twenty years ago.

A recent study from UCLA estimated that 46 percent of the adult population in California currently has prediabetes or undiagnosed diabetes, including 33 percent of those eighteen to thirty-nine years old. Another 9 percent have already been diagnosed with diabetes. This is a stunning 55 percent (well over half) of the state's population. Most of the prediabetics will go on to type 2 diabetes, and many will ultimately suffer from chronic and non-healing wounds and all of the other horrible complications of diabetes. Another recent study from the UK noted that childhood cancer rates in Britain have risen 40 percent in the past ten years. This, despite all of the amazing technological advances in medicine. What is going on?

Driven by my usual curiosity and an insatiable desire to improve my own health and aging process, I started again asking "Why?" I have since realized that much of what we do in the modern mainstream medical system is to serve as marketing arm of the pharmaceutical companies (and you would not believe the cost of some chemotherapy drugs).

Realizing my formal training was lacking, I pursued fellowship training in anti-aging and regenerative medicine (A4M) and age management medicine. There I was introduced to the importance of the hormonal and nutritional milieu in which our bodies operate and the concept that the body knows how to heal itself if we can just create the right conditions. Following my instincts to delve deeper into the actual roots of health and disease, I began to study even more esoteric subjects, such as light, quantum physics and biology, chronobiology, electromagnetic fields, and other fields of "alternative" medicine. Dr. Jack Kruse taught me that precepts of quantum physics actually apply to our biology. I have learned about the importance of energy flows and mitochondria in health and disease.

During my fellowship in stem cell therapy, I had been amazed by the success we can achieve by moving these important cells from one part of the body to another, activating them with the body's own growth factors, and letting them go to work decreasing pain, restoring function, and rebuilding the target tissues. It is an example of how the body, with a little assistance from doctors, really can heal itself.

One essential truth I have learned during my quest for knowledge is that *nature is the best physician*. The word "doctor" comes from the Latin *Docere*, which means "to educate," and the most important part of my role as a physician is to help educate my patients about the natural healing processes of their amazing bodies. Our bodies have the knowledge, the wisdom, and the capability of healing when we create the right conditions, give them the right nutrients and substrates, give them access to the right energies and light, and then get out of the way.

WHY WRITE A BOOK ABOUT WOUNDS?

What do two married doctors talk about in the evenings after our three children are in bed, the seven dogs are fed, and the kitchen is cleaned? We compare stories about our patients, our days, and our frustrations with the current healthcare system. We realize that we can help many more people heal, and heal faster. Millions worldwide are needlessly suffering from chronic wounds and undergoing amputations.

By combining the expertise of a wound care physician with the advanced and alternative techniques and knowledge from the specialty of anti-aging and regenerative medicine, we open new possibilities to exponentially improve healing. We have created a revolutionary wound care program in which we optimize your wound and body's environment for healing and provide teachings from nature, not just for healing your wound but also for healing your body.

Many of the things we discuss are well outside the tunnel vision of traditional mainstream medicine and thus are not practiced at wound care centers. Most doctors and even top universities know nothing about some of the methods we discuss—because they are not going to fill the pockets of pharmaceutical companies, insurance companies, and hospitals.

Many of the techniques and methods we have developed do not require a specialized wound center but rather knowledge, motivation, effort, and lifestyle changes. We will describe many things you and your loved ones can do at home for better health. A chronic and non-healing wound is a sign of a stressed and sick body, and the best place to start healing your wound is by healing *you*.

In our day-to-day practices, we touch one life at a time. We want to share what we have learned with *anyone* who has a non-healing wound, as well as caregivers and other healthcare providers. If you or a loved one has a wound that is healing slowly, poorly, or not at all, know that there are millions of others like you, and *there is help*. Embrace today as the day you regain your *hope* for healing.

CHAPTER 1

Don't Let Them Take Your Leg!

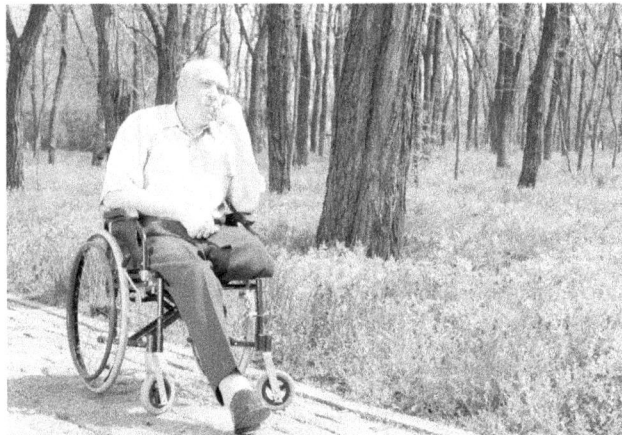

Case Report from Dr. Rob Hamilton

A few years ago, while working a shift in the emergency department, I took care of Mrs. T, a fifty-six year-old woman. She had just been discharged from the hospital earlier in the day after having a below the knee amputation (BKA). Only two hours after arriving home, she had tried to stand up from a chair that she was sitting in, and forgetting that she no longer had a leg on the right side, she had fallen and hit the end of her stump, causing it to bleed. Fortunately, the injury was minor, and we ultimately were able to discharge her after discussing her care with the orthopedist who had taken her leg off.

Curious, I had asked her more about what had led to her amputation. She had been a type 2 diabetic for several years and had developed neuropathy (a lack of feeling in her legs). A few months earlier, she had gotten an infection in her big toe (it became red and swollen) after accidentally trimming her toenail too close to the skin. Despite being placed on antibiotics by her primary medical doctor (PMD), the infection worsened and she was admitted to the hospital and placed on IV antibiotics. There was little improvement, so an orthopedic surgeon was consulted. He recommended amputation of the toe.

Sadly, she agreed to proceed because the orthopedist told her there was no other option, and her PMD and the hospitalist (doctor taking care of her in the hospital) agreed. After her toe was amputated, she was discharged from the hospital on antibiotics.

Despite the antibiotics, the wound from her toe amputation never closed and continued to drain. When she followed up with the orthopedist a few weeks later, he told her that it was unlikely that the wound was going to ever heal, so he recommended a transmetatarsal amputation. This is basically cutting off most of the foot. Her PMD once again agreed and told her it was the only reasonable course of action. She agreed to proceed.

After the transmetatarsal amputation, once again her wound did not heal well. This is not surprising, as diabetics have markedly impaired circulation and healing capacity and frequently need a lot of special techniques to help heal their wounds. She continued to have drainage, and no new skin grew to cover the raw, ulcerated areas.

Once again, after additional follow-up visits to the orthopedist and despite antibiotics, she was told that the wound from the trans-metatarsal amputation would never heal and the only option left for her was a BKA. (After a BKA, about a quarter of the lower leg below the knee is left with the hope that the patient can learn to walk with a prosthesis.) Again, her PMD agreed and advised her to go ahead with it.

Her BKA was three days prior to the time I saw her and, of course, that led to her visiting the ER. I suspected this would be the first of many times she would have a problem with her stump; it is well known to doctors that many BKA patients end up with pressure ulcers, sores, and infections on the end of their stump, even those with the best-fitting prosthetic legs.

I asked her if she had ever been referred to our local wound care center, and she told me that she had never heard of a wound care center. She had not even been told such an option was available. This was frustrating to me as the wound center has been open for eight years, has taken care of thousands of patients of nearly every doctor in the community, and actively markets what they do. I know because my wife lectures frequently in the community about the wound center and talks to many of the doctors (including the orthopedist who recommended the progressive amputations). I did not know whether her doctors just did not know of the option (unlikely) or did not think it would help (more likely but absolutely wrong).

I discussed the case that night with Dr. Julie, who explained that, unfortunately, she hears stories like this all the time from her patients. Many patients undergo an amputation before ever getting referred to a wound center. Sometimes she gets involved after only the initial toe or transmetatarsal amputation (and can still fight to save the rest of the leg). But sometimes she never has an opportunity to intervene until a patient's surgical above- or below-knee amputation stump will not heal after surgery, and then the orthopedic surgeon has nothing else to offer and finally sends the patient to the wound center (there is nothing left to amputate).

I am certain that, had Mrs. T gone to the wound care center, she would never have even had her big toe amputated. Instead, she just kept seeing her orthopedist and her primary care physician who continued to recommend that the orthopedist serially cut off portions of her leg, leaving her functionally crippled for the rest of her life.

I felt terrible for Mrs. T, who told me she had to take weeks off work to recover from each of the amputations. She still wants to watch her grandchildren's soccer games and travel. I knew she might never get a prosthesis and learn to walk normally, or even if she could walk with it, she would be at increased risks for falls and other injury. I knew she would never be able to hike, walk on the beach, or walk on rough or uneven surfaces again. Even getting up the few stairs into her home creates huge effort and risk. She is now handicapped for life. That loss of mobility detracts significantly from happiness, mood, and lifespan. I knew she would ultimately suffer from depression and frustration, especially if she ever discovered how unnecessary the BKA might have been.

In addition, I knew the mortality statistics after amputation. Although amputation may sometimes be necessary, *it should absolutely be considered the last resort.* The rapid, sequential nibbling away of someone's body, mobility, and independence should not be taken lightly, and all other options should be exhausted first.

Do not let them take your leg—at least not without a fight. Do everything you can to avoid it!

AMPUTATION DRASTICALLY CHANGES YOUR LIFE

Imagine what it is like to have to face an amputation, or perhaps you are facing one now and feeling worried and anxious about it—with good reason.

Not only do those who have an amputation have to significantly adjust their lifestyle and get used to living in a wheelchair or getting around with either a prosthetic limb or crutches, but they are also at a substantially greater risk for falls and other injuries. It is truly debilitating.

All of us who took those first stumbling steps as toddlers then learned to walk and run take that ability for granted. That easy bipedal mobility is part of our natural skill set as humans. If you want to get up and walk across the room to the bathroom or to get a glass of water, it is easy. Most of us can unconsciously transition from lying or sitting to standing and walking without

Learning to walk on a prosthesis

even thinking about it. Try to imagine—if you can—how different it would be

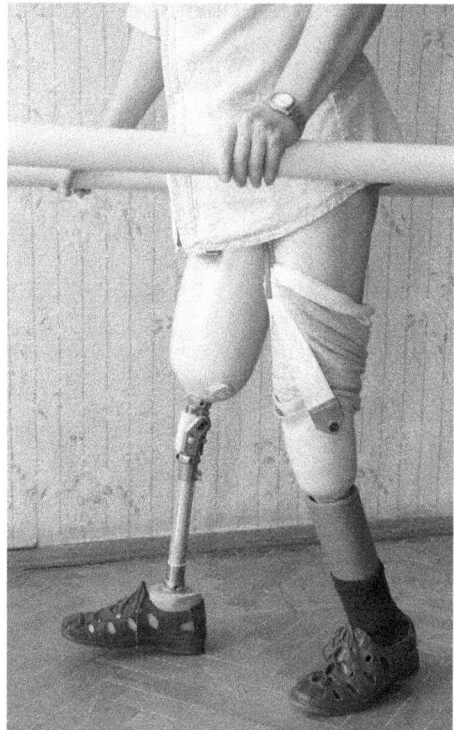

if you were confined to a wheelchair or bed and could not just spring up at a moment's notice to take a few steps to get what you wanted or needed.

Even if you have mastered "walking and chewing gum at the same time," realize that mastering walking with a prosthesis requires a whole different level of skill and training. Even if you have a well-fitting prosthesis, every step takes a different kind of strength and balance than you have ever had to muster, and it takes time to develop and change yourself so that it feels natural. You will have to think carefully about every step and movement, and if wheelchair-bound, just getting out of your wheelchair into a car, or onto a couch, or onto a toilet, or into bed necessitates a complex series of movements and transfers that you may not even be able to do without assistance. There goes your freedom, your independence, and unfortunately all too often your self-respect and happiness.

After an amputation, it becomes difficult or impossible to climb or descend stairs or go for walks. You may lose your ability to drive yourself or may need to spend tens of thousands of dollars for a specially outfitted vehicle, and you will need to outfit your home with ramps and rails. Many people with amputations also develop pressure ulcers from ill-fitting prosthetics. Others do not have the strength or balance to walk with a prosthesis and end up wheelchair bound. For some, this necessitates moving from their home into a nursing facility or assisted living with the attendant drastic decrease in quality of life. It can be financially devastating as the cost of care goes up, and ability to work may be drastically reduced or completely eradicated.

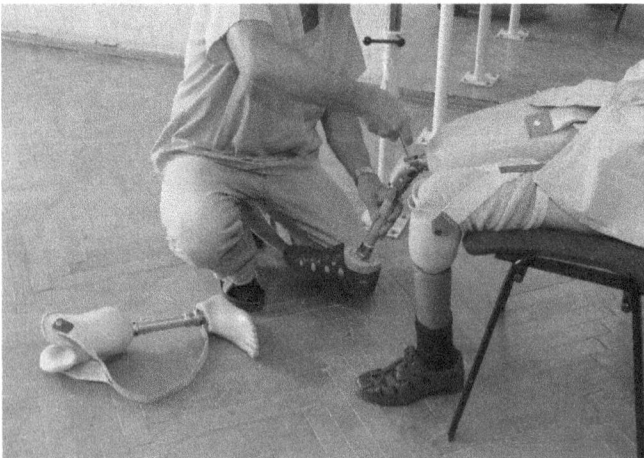

Although we have the utmost respect for those

who have had to adapt and are able to successfully navigate their new lives on a prosthesis or in a wheelchair—and we know and have taken care of many, we also know that it does not necessarily have to be this way. We urge you to make sure it is the absolute last resort and make sure to do everything you can and seek out the right care to help you avoid this.

AMPUTATION DRASTICALLY SHORTENS YOUR LIFE

Most people do not realize that an amputation does not only affect quality but also affects their quantity (length) of life. We do not think many of the surgeons performing those amputations realize that the average risk of dying after a lower extremity amputation within the next five years is greater than 50 percent.

In fact, some believe that the 50 percent mortality statistic may even underestimate the risk. A 2008 article in the *Journal of American Podiatry Medical Association* entitled "Mortality Rates and Diabetic Foot Ulcers. Is it Time to Communicate Mortality Risk to Patients with Diabetic Foot Ulceration?" Here is a summary of the findings:

- Five-year death rates after new-onset diabetic ulceration have been reported to be between 43 percent and 55 percent.

- Five-year death rates were as high as 74 percent for patients who underwent lower-extremity amputation.

These rates are higher than those for several types of cancer including prostate, breast, colon, and Hodgkin's disease. These alarmingly high five-year mortality rates need to be addressed and patients need to be made aware of the seriousness of having a wound *and* diabetes. Providers and patients alike must realize that any new-onset diabetic foot ulcer must be urgently managed. All too often these patients slowly work their way through the system before they eventually (if ever) get referred to a wound care center, or the "aggressive man-agement" just turns out to be aggressive amputation with resultant lifetime disability (and increased mortality) as in the case of Mrs. T.

New-onset diabetic foot ulcers should be considered a marker for significantly increased mortality.

While it can be argued whether or not the five-year mortality after ampu-tation is due to the amputation itself, or the need for amputation is just an indicator of poor health and severity of underlying disease, it is absolutely certain that any diabetic foot ulcer (frankly any type of chronic wound) must be taken very seriously.

A vibrantly healthy person does not develop or harbor a chronic wound; a chronic wound is an indicator of ill health. Unfortunately, the concomitant inflammation and infection that occurs with a chronic wound contributes even more to worsening health. This creates a vicious circle from which it takes a lot of effort, knowledge, and care to escape. As we have mentioned, even the wound center cannot heal every wound or save every limb, but they have a much better chance of doing it than you will find elsewhere.

Mrs. T's experience shows the limitations and failings of current main-stream medicine. Another patient who had three different doctors recommend-ing an amputation while in the hospital refused because she had seen Dr. Julie once and had the confidence and knowledge to "just say no." Unfortunately, Mrs. T and countless others were not referred to a wound center where the outcome might have been very different.

If you are committed to healing and willing to embrace some of the knowledge we share, seek out the right care (whether at a local wound center and other appropriate practitioners), and make some important lifestyle changes, you *can* heal. You will not only heal your chronic wound but also vastly improve your health and escape becoming one of those awful mortality statistics. We want to help you break that cycle, improve your health, heal that wound, and live your life to its fullest without the pain, inconvenience, stigma, or misery of losing your leg.

Live your best life possible! Fight for your leg!

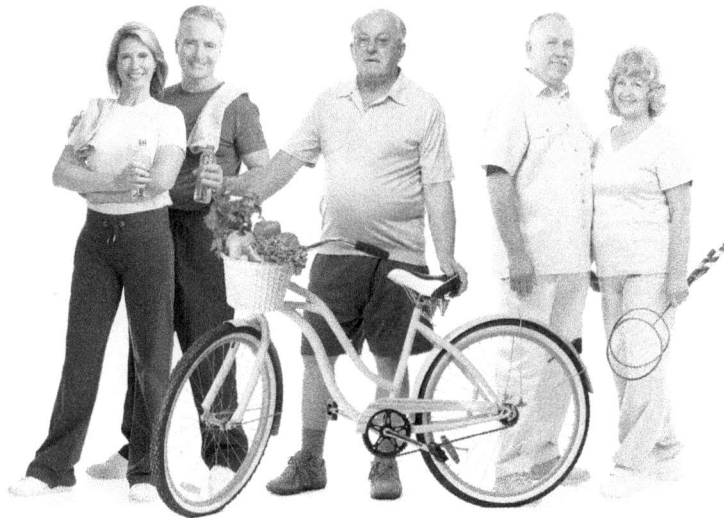

References and Recommended Reading

1. "Depression and Wound Healing." *Advanced Tissue*. Advanced Tissue, 27 Jan. 2016. Web. 11 June 2017.

2. Robbins, JM, et al. "Mortality Rates and Diabetic Foot Ulcers. Is it Time to Communicate Mortality Risk to Patients with Diabetic Foot Ulceration?" *J of Am Podiatry Med Assoc*, 98 (6): 489-493, 2008.

3. CDC. National Diabetes Statistics Report: Estimates of Diabetes and Its Burden in the United States, 2014. Atlanta, GA: US Dept of Health and Human Services; 2014

4. Nguyen, Benjamin. "Don't Laugh: I Just Want to Help My Patients." *KevinMD*. KevinMD, 13 Jan. 2017. Web. 11 June 2017.

5. Bolton L. "Evidence Corner: Exploring Social Isolation of Leg Ulcer Patients." *WOUNDS* 2017;29(4):122–124.

CHAPTER 2

The Diabetes Apocalypse

Over the last few years in the United States, movies and television shows depicting a so-called "zombie apocalypse" have become increasingly popular. You may not realize it, but the world is now facing a much more expensive and lethal epidemic—a diabetes apocalypse! For the first time in decades, our life expectancy has declined, and studies suggest that type 2 diabetes is a major factor.

Until recently, diabetes was considered the seventh leading cause of death in the United States. Now experts believe that it is probably the third leading cause of death after cancer and heart disease. Diabetes will be directly responsible for the death of eight million people this year worldwide.

In 1985, approximately thirty million people worldwide had diabetes. Between 1990 and 2013, diabetes rates rose by 71 percent in the United States. With obesity on the rise, millions more are at risk of developing diabetes. By

2030, according to the World Health Organization, at least 366 million are projected to have diabetes. This is frankly astounding, and the number is not at all proportional to the population increase.

"The rise in obesity has hit the United States hard. More than a third of adults and one-fifth of children and adolescents age 2 to 19 are obese."

—*Harvard Gazette*, May 3, 2017

Here are a few more grim facts regarding the incidence of type 2 diabetes (T2D) in the United States:

- Every day in the United States, approximately five thousand people are diagnosed with T2D.

- 8.1 million Americans with diabetes are unaware of their disease.

- A recent UCLA study estimated 46 percent of the population of California is prediabetic—they are only a few years from developing diabetes—9 percent already have it.

- The CDC estimates that eighty-two million Americans will have T2D by the end of 2026, and one in three adults will have T2D by 2050.

About one out of three people with type 2 diabetes do not know they have it because early symptoms are mild or they have not been tested.

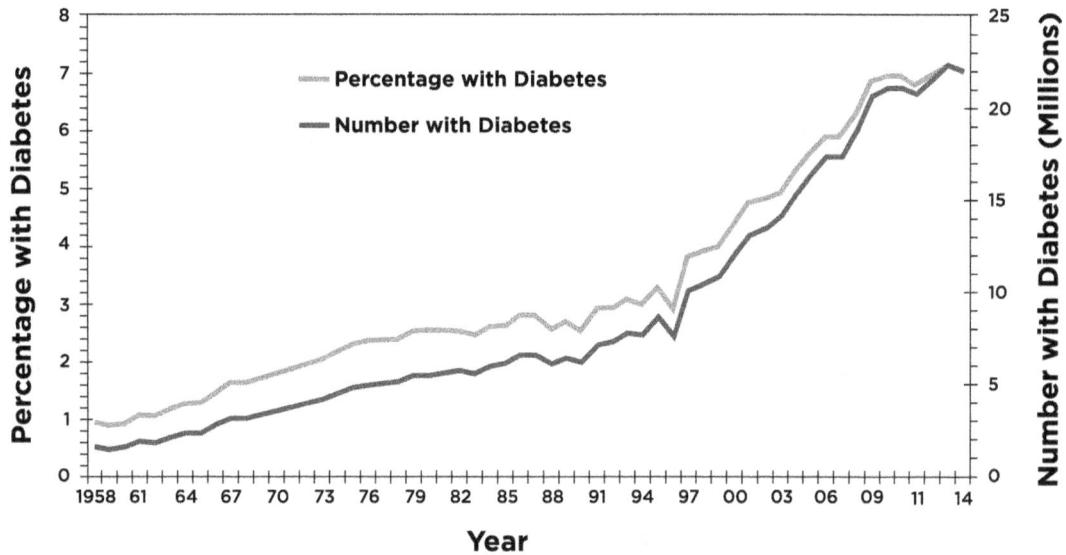

Source: Centers for Disease Control and Prevention (CDC), "Long-Term Trends in Diabetes," April 2016. Americans diagnosed with diabetes, 1958 through 2014.

T2D used to be referred to as "adult onset diabetes mellitus" when we were in medical school (not that long ago) and was considered a disease of the elderly (seventies and eighties). It is now routinely diagnosed in people in their twenties and thirties and even in teenagers and children. Recently, a three-year-old girl in Texas was diagnosed with T2D. We all recognize the relationship between diet, lack of exercise, and obesity with T2D, but despite awareness and a focus by doctors and public health officials on prevention, the incidence continues to rise.

T2D is entirely preventable and in most cases reversible. We will discuss other factors, such as the light environment we now live in, which have been linked to this rapidly increasing disease. We will present new ways to help you reverse T2D.

WHAT IS DIABETES ANYWAY?

Most of you know that *diabetes mellitus* is characterized by having a high blood sugar level. "Diabetes mellitus" actually means "sweet urine" as previous generations of doctors used to diagnose it by tasting the urine of patients. They noted that people with diabetes had sweet urine, as the excess sugar in their bloodstream was excreted in the urine. Fortunately, we now have laboratory blood and urine tests that can diagnose it without that level of physician involvement.

If untreated, high blood sugar levels can lead to all kinds of complications, including an impaired immune system (more infections), dysfunction of nerves (neuropathy), which can either be very painful or result in loss of feeling in your limbs, kidney disease or outright kidney failure, blindness, and a host of other problems. T2D substantially increases the risk of cardiovascular disease (heart attacks), strokes, and dementia (think Alzheimer's disease). This excess glucose in turn leads to physiological effects such as hypoxia in the cells. Prolonged and persistent oxygen shortage for a cell means the cell goes into a death spiral, functioning ever more poorly. The person is no longer able to perform at normal levels, vitality is sapped, and chronic ailments set in.

Diabetes increases your risk for heart disease, blindness, nerve and organ damage, and amputations. It strikes people of all ages.

The exact mechanisms by which diabetes causes these problems in different organ systems is very complex. One simplistic mechanism is thought to be that the excess sugar floating around in the bloodstream binds to various proteins in the body (a process called glycosylation) and that glycosylated proteins are like rust or corrosion on the inside of pipes. They are dysfunctional and stick to things and places that they should not. The more your body corrodes internally, the more rapidly you age and the more diseases you acquire. Chronically elevated insulin levels in the blood as your body tries to deal with the excess sugar also lead to other metabolic problems that compound the damage.

Diabetes is generally classified by doctors as two … well … now three types:

1. Type 1 diabetes, also called "insulin dependent diabetes," was previously called "juvenile diabetes." This is an autoimmune disease afflicting more than two hundred thousand Americans per year and the numbers are climbing. In this type, the pancreas, an abdominal organ that secretes insulin (and other digestive enzymes and some hormones) for some reason (usually thought to be autoimmune), stops producing insulin. Insulin is a critical hormone that helps move glucose (sugar) out of the bloodstream and into the cells where it is used to help produce the energy you need to go about your daily life. These patients must take exogenous insulin, usually by injection or a pump, in order to be able to transport glucose into their cells. Without insulin, their cells cannot make use of the energy, and they develop a very high glucose level in the blood.

2. Type 2 diabetes (T2D), previously referred to as "adult onset" diabetes, is characterized by insulin resistance. Unlike type 1, in T2D the pancreas has been producing so much insulin for so long that the other cells in the body such as (primarily but not only) muscle cells stop being responsive to the insulin, either by decreasing the number of insulin receptors on their cell surfaces, or just not being able to produce enough insulin receptors to transport all the overwhelming amount of glucose in the bloodstream into the cells.

   The ultimate result is that the pancreas cannot produce enough insulin to cope with all the glucose in the bloodstream. There are many different pathways that are targeted by the various medications used to treat T2D, although sometimes medications are not enough and patients must resort to insulin, which actually can worsen the disease process which is caused by insulin resistance to start with. Some patients and even misinformed healthcare providers refer to type 2 diabetics who take insulin as "insulin dependent diabetics," but note that their disease has a very different basis than that of type 1 diabetics, who truly are dependent on exogenous insulin just to live. It is T2D that is exploding in prevalence.

Diabetics are more likely to develop plaque in their arteries, which slows blood flow and increases risk of clots. It leads to hardening of the arteries (called atherosclerosis), which increases the risk of heart attack, stroke, and poor blood flow to the feet and legs. Even small foot sores can develop gangrene and infection. Combine this with diabetic nerve damage, which makes it hard to feel your feet. Wounds may go unnoticed until there is drainage and odor, signifying that an infection has already set in.

3. Type 3 diabetes, just starting to be recognized as a medical condition by researchers, is insulin resistance in the brain, and it leads to dementia (think Alzheimer's disease). When the brain has been exposed to high blood sugars for too long and becomes insulin resistant, eventually it cannot use the available glucose to produce the energy required for thinking, memory, decision-making, controlling the various organ systems, and all the other processes that characterize a healthy brain.

DIABETES AND WOUNDS

Diabetes is a major cause of lack of circulation and feeling in the lower limbs, which predisposes to ulcerations. Diabetic foot ulcers all too often end in amputations, and as in the case of Mrs. T in Chapter 2, they frequently do not stop with just the affected toe or the forefoot, but often end up with BKAs (below-knee amputations). Did you know that every hour, ten Americans undergo an amputation due to diabetes?

It is estimated that up to 85 percent of all amputations due to diabetes could (should?) have been prevented.

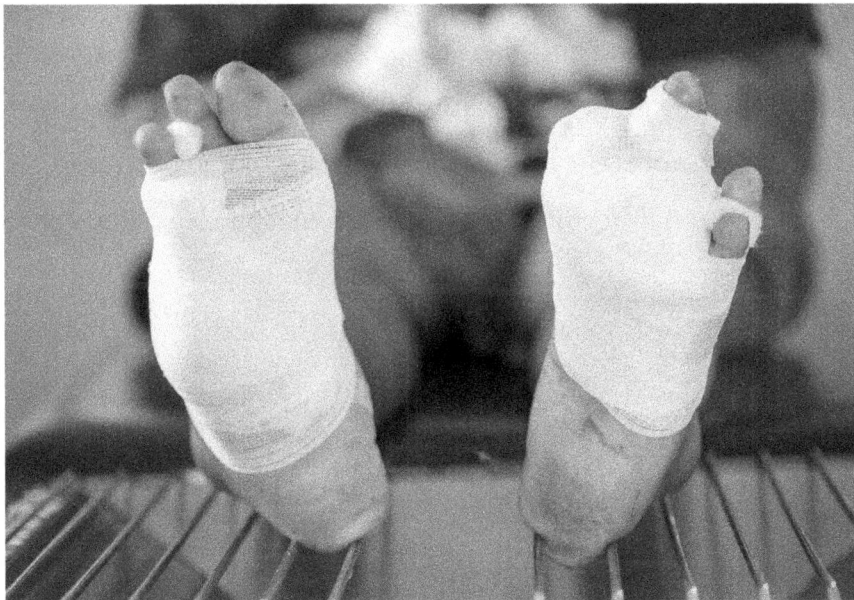

Chronic ulcers are caused by diabetes for several reasons:

1. Diabetes causes both macrovascular (large blood vessel) and microvascular (small blood vessel) disease. This compromises blood

flow to the leg and foot, which means limited delivery of oxygen, healing-type cells, and immune modulators.

2. Chronically high blood sugars cause glycosylation of proteins that end up "clogging" blood vessels, both large and small, and impairing the ability of the body to get blood where it needs to promote healing. This is particularly true in the legs and feet. The farther one gets from the heart the more this affects the blood flow. Now you know why the most common and stubbornly difficult to heal diabetic wounds (and the most common amputations) are on the toes.

3. In addition to clogging and making blood vessels dysfunctional, diabetes impairs the body's immune system function. Your immune system is constantly working to protect your body from a variety of bacteria, viruses, and other pathological agents. Once the immune system is impaired and the blood flow is constricted, it becomes very difficult to heal chronic wounds, particularly on the legs or feet. The skin is an important barrier against infection, so non-intact skin and a dysfunctional immune system mean that the legs or feet of diabetics are at a tremendously high risk for infection, which can quickly spread to the bone or unchecked throughout the body.

4. Diabetes also causes neuropathy, which is a condition that diminishes nerve function. The exact mechanism is unclear, but again, the farther away from the heart and central circulation, the more likely neuropathy is. Diabetic patients with neuropathy often either lose the feeling in their legs and feet or occasionally have severe pain (it is miserable). Once a person loses the ability to feel their feet and legs, even small scratches and wounds that normal people get every day can quickly turn into very serious and even life-threatening problems before they are noticed. Because of the neuropathy, infection may not

cause pain, so it is very important to diligently inspect all surfaces of the feet and legs frequently. Oftentimes the wounds are only noticed when they become very large or difficult to treat. To illustrate just how quickly this can happen, we will share a few cases with you.

Case Reports from Dr. Julie Hamilton

- Mr. H is a sixty-one-year-old veteran with T2D who developed an ulcer on the bottom of his foot from ill-fitting shoes. He was treated at the VA clinic and reported that "iodine paste" had been used on his wound "for weeks." He woke up one day and his entire foot was red and swollen so he went to the ER. He was admitted with a diabetic foot infection and started on IV antibiotics. I consulted the next day and drained the abscess, which had developed in the bottom of his foot. When I probed the draining tract in the space between his first and second metatarsals, my sterile curette came right out the top of his foot. He was convinced that he was going to lose his leg as so many of his friends had. After continued IV antibiotics along with weekly visits to the wound center and eventually hyperbaric oxygen treatments (HBOT) as well, Mr. H went on to heal his wound with no loss of toes, forefoot, or lower leg. He is thrilled that he can still walk and drive his Corvette.

- Mrs. V is a seventy-two-year-old woman with T2D who was visiting her daughter. While walking barefoot across the wood floor, she thinks she snagged her toe on a splinter. She felt nothing but noticed blood on the floor. She applied antibiotic ointment and a Band-Aid. Two days later, she looked down and the toe was red and swollen, and there was a red streak moving up her foot. She started taking clindamycin ("I had some leftover in my purse from a dental procedure") and said the red streak went away, but the open wound never healed (got worse) and her toe still looked red. When she returned home, her nurse practitioner prescribed another antibiotic and referred her to a podiatrist. He instructed her to soak her toe in Epsom salt and warm water. Gradually her wound turned dark, dry, and more painful. She finally saw the podiatrist two to three weeks later. By this time, she had a Grade 3 ulcer (deep space infection beneath the black eschar), and the podiatrist appropriately referred her to the wound center. She eventually healed with debridement, offloading, biologic products, and HBOT.

- Mr. S is an active fifty-four-year-old without medical problems (or a primary doctor) who liked to walk his German shepherds two to three miles a day. "I pulled a callus off the tip of my big toe one day, and it bled." He dressed it daily after soaking his foot in Epsom salt and warm water. He thought it was getting better because it stopped oozing and bleeding, but it "turned black." He tried to get a doctor's appointment, which was scheduled in two months. Two weeks later, his toe became more painful, red, and swollen. He went to the ER and was admitted with a necrotic, infected toe. He was found to have a very high blood sugar (undiagnosed T2D) and neuropathy. The infection had already spread to the bone (osteomyelitis). The orthopedic surgeon recommended (and performed) amputation of his big toe. He was discharged on insulin and antibiotics, and his surgical wound eventually healed. Several weeks later, he noticed a foul-smelling callus on the second toe "but I remembered they told me never to pull off a callus," so he kept a Band-Aid in place. Weeks later "the dead skin fell off" and he noticed "a deep hole." By this time, he had a primary physician who referred him to the wound center. His wound was found to tunnel down to the bone; a bone culture was taken. The osteomyelitis had spread. I prescribed appropriate antibiotics and kept pressure off his toe with a specialized shoe. He was eventually authorized by his insurance to start HBOT, and his wound healed with no further amputations. He will always require a custom-molded filler inside his shoe to prevent sliding and further injury due to loss of his big toe.

• Mrs. H is a sixty-two-year-old woman with diabetes who made the mistake of riding her stationary bicycle wearing socks only. She only pedaled for fifteen minutes, but shortly after getting off, noticed that her left heel had a large, fluid-filled blister from rubbing against the heel strap. It took three weeks to see her doctor and get a referral to our wound center. By this time, the wound had ulcerated and become foul-smelling and necrotic. It took months of aggressive treatment, revascularization, off-loading, and HBOT to finally heal.

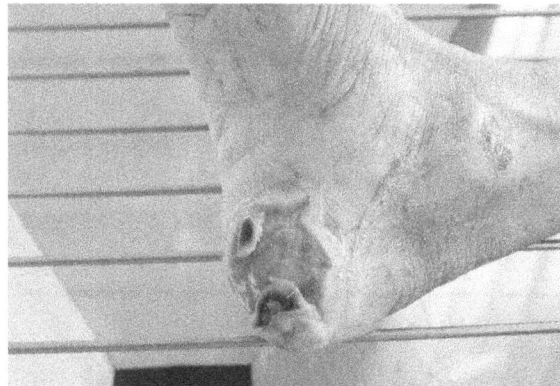

JUST SAY NO!

Twenty-five percent of diabetics will develop a non-healing wound over their lifetime and approximately 15 percent will eventually end up with an amputation. In addition, 27 percent will undergo a second amputation within one year of their first amputation. We have seen this scenario play out many times; it is *so* critical to avoid that first amputation if possible.

People do not realize (and are not told) that if a surgeon removes "only" your big toe, your foot will never be the same. The weight-bearing load now transfers to the other toes and footpad, deformities gradually develop in the other toes (hammertoe deformities, etc.) and metatarsal bones, and calluses occur. You will require custom orthotics or boots just to be able to walk without developing another wound. Even worse, as we have already discussed, up to 74 percent of patients die within five years of their first amputation. This cycle must be stopped before it starts.

Death rates for diabetic foot ulcers (DFUs) and the accompanying amputations are higher than for many cancers, including breast cancer, prostate cancer, and Hodgkin's lymphoma.

Here are a few more sobering facts about diabetes, wounds, and amputations:

- Eighty-five percent of diabetes-related lower leg amputations are preceded by a foot ulcer.

- More than one million diabetics in the United States have had amputations.

- Approximately eighty-five thousand amputations are performed every year in the United States.

- Every day in the United States, diabetes accounts for about two hundred lives lost and more than two hundred limbs amputated.

- A limb is amputated in the United States every six minutes and every twenty seconds worldwide.

Most non-healing wounds last on average twelve to thirteen months, and if they heal at all, they recur in up to 60 to 70 percent of patients (an indicator of their poor health).

Advanced treatment at a wound center should be considered early—actually, immediately—and viewed as the standard of care, not as a last resort. The goal in treating DFUs is prompt and complete healing. The longer the wound exists, the harder to heal and the greater likelihood it will lead to serious complications, amputations, and an ever-tightening spiral of worsening chronic illness. A diabetic ulcer is a race against time to save your limb.

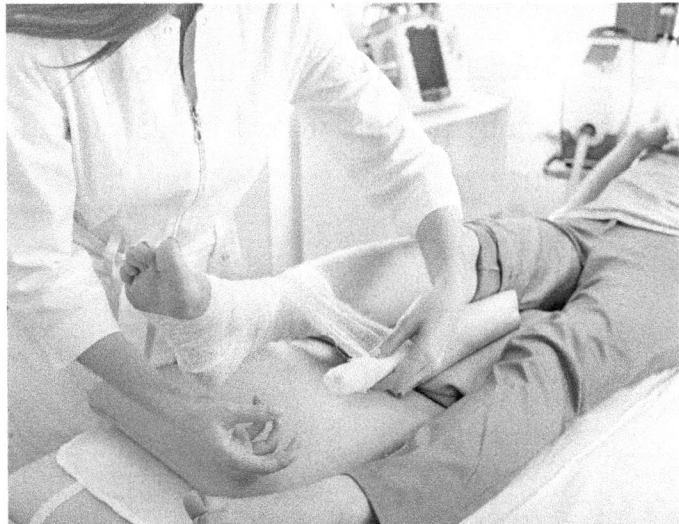

References and Recommended Reading

1. www.CDC.gov

2. Smith A, "Guidelines-Based Screening May Miss Up to Half of Diabetic and Prediabetic Patients." *MD Magazine*. August 2016, 6 (5): 7.

3. Mercola, Joseph. "Diabetes Has Become One of the Most Expensive and Lethal Diseases in the World." *Mercola.com*. Dr. Mercola. Web. 11 June 2017.

4. Driver V., et al. "Health Economic Implications for Wound Care and Limb Preservation." *J Managed Care Med*. 2008, 11(1): 13–19.

5. "Statistics About Diabetes." *Diabetes.org*. American Diabetes Association. Web. 11 June 2017.

6. Mercola, Joseph. "How Sugar Harms Your Brains Health and Drives the Alzheimer's Epidemic." *Mercola.com*. Dr. Mercola, 24 July 2014. Web. 11 June 2017.

7. Gallagher KA et al. "Epigenetic Changes in Bone Marrow Progenitor Cells Influence the Inflammatory Phenotype and Alter Wound Healing in Type 2 Diabetes." *Diabetes* 2015 Apr: 64 (4): 1420–1430.

8. Fife CE, Carter MJ, et al. "Wound care outcomes and associated cost among patients treated in US outpatient wound centers." *Wounds*. 2012;24(1).

CHAPTER 3

With Diabetes, Even a Scratch Can Kill

Given the prevalence of diabetes and the number of non-healing diabetic wounds, we want to focus on a few important things you should know. With diabetes, even minor wounds can quickly turn serious or even life threatening. The best treatment is prevention.

Many diabetics have neuropathy (nerve damage) in their feet so they have no feeling. Their feet are numb.

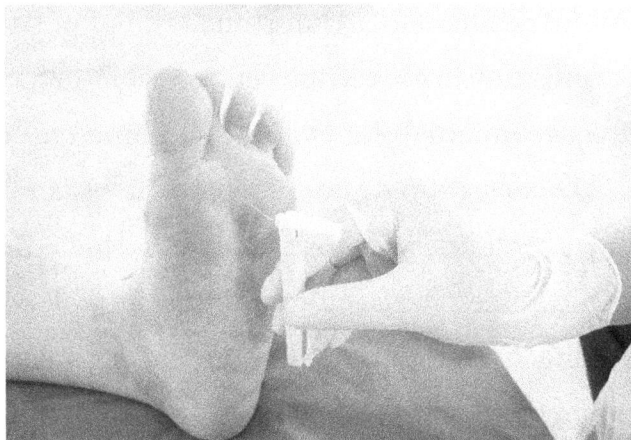

Monofilament testing for presence of sensation—performed on the first visit to our wound center

Sensations of pain, discomfort, heat, or pressure are either significantly reduced or absent. There is a two-minute test that can be done at wound centers to evaluate for the presence of neuropathy.

Intact nerves tell most of us if we have a blister, cut, or callus on our foot, but diabetics have no such warning symptoms. They develop foot ulcers simply from pressure walking in new or tight-fitting shoes or having a small pebble stuck in their shoe. They may blister from friction or walking barefoot on hot surfaces. They develop cuts from sand rubbing between their toes while walking on the beach in flip-flops. They get puncture wounds from walking barefoot, even inside their homes. We have seen all of these scenarios—repeatedly.

THE DANGERS OF DIABETES

If you have diabetes, you are at particular risk for infection, and it is critical that you clean all wounds thoroughly, watch them carefully as they heal, and seek help immediately if you have any concerns for infection at all—usually signified by worsening pain, redness, drainage (particularly pus), puffiness, swelling, fevers, chills, joint aches, your blood sugar getting out of control, or even just feeling poorly. Even seemingly benign infections can penetrate to muscle and bone. Unfortunately, if you have neuropathy, it is possible that an infection may become quite severe before being recognized. Once bone becomes infected these wounds become very challenging to heal.

Diabetes also causes blood vessel walls to thicken and become less elastic (peripheral artery disease or PAD). This especially affects the smaller vessels of the ankles, feet, and toes. Decreased blood flow obviously impairs wound healing. Even routine scrapes and blisters may worsen very quickly and develop gangrene. Smokers are also at significant risk for PAD (diabetics who smoke are nearly guaranteed to have it).

There is a ten-minute test that we perform at wound centers on the very first visit to screen patients for PAD. If abnormal, further evaluation with ultrasound or angiography is scheduled. This may lead to angioplasty (inflating a balloon inside the diseased artery) and stenting (deploying a little "scaffold" to keep a constricted artery open to blood flow). If that fails, a vascular surgeon may be needed to perform a bypass procedure, where the artery above the blockage is connected to one of the arteries in the calf. Unless ischemia is treated aggressively, an ulcer may develop gangrene and result in limb amputation.

Another serious problem that diabetics face is bone infection (osteomyelitis). Signs include bone pain, fever, chills, excessive sweating, swelling (sometimes of the entire extremity), redness, drainage, and pain at the infection site. If a wound can be probed all the way to bone, it is presumed that osteomyelitis is present. If purulent drainage creates an opening at the site of a previously healed wound or fracture, osteomyelitis is likely. Diabetic foot ulcers that fail to heal (or reoccur for no other obvious reason) often have underlying osteomyelitis as the cause. Chronic osteomyelititis is especially hard to treat.

Some clinical tests to evaluate for osteomyelitis include labs (such as ESR, C-reactive protein, and increased platelets with decreased serum albumin), bone biopsies and cultures, bone scans, x-rays, and magnetic resonance imaging (MRI). If a doctor suspects that a patient may have a bone infection, it is important to obtain diagnostic tests so that aggressive treatment may begin as soon as possible.

Treatment for osteomyelitis involves resolving the infection through a combination of surgery, IV antibiotic therapy, and excellent wound care. Hyperbaric oxygen therapy (HBOT) is typically only authorized by

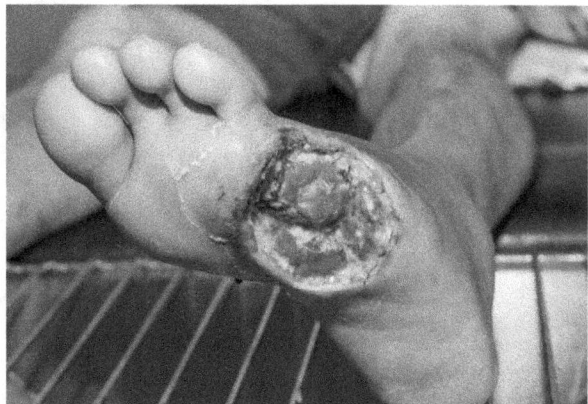

insurance companies and other payers in cases of chronic and refractory osteo-myelitis. Osteomyelitis can sometimes be treated successfully with oral antibi-otics but usually removal of the infected bone is necessary.

If there is infection surrounding screws, plates, or pins in bone (usually placed for joint replacement or fracture repair), the hardware must be removed to resolve the infection. Bone grafts with antibiotics may be inserted to fill in the spaces left by the removal of dead bone and to encourage the growth of new bone. HBOT is also very beneficial.

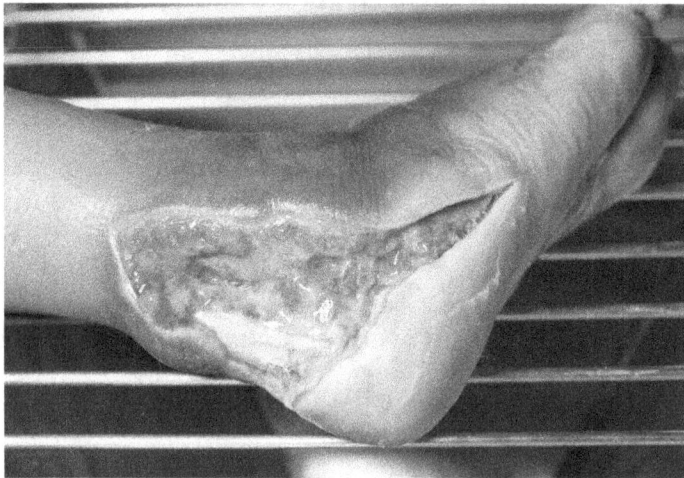

WOUND PREVENTION IS KEY

1. Tight glucose control is critical for both type 1 and type 2 diabetics, especially when trying to heal a wound. Glycosylated hemoglobin, known as Hemoglobin A1C (HbA1C) is the most useful marker of recent control (goal < 5.7 percent). Glycemic control is a reflection of many other metabolic processes.

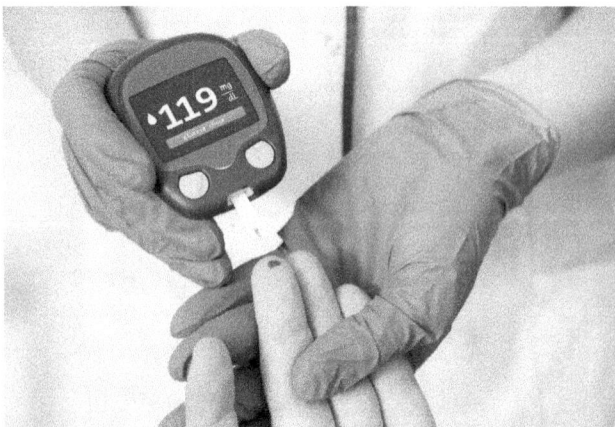

2. Inspect your feet daily. If you have lost feeling in your feet, look to see if anything is wrong *every* time you remove your shoes.

3. Wash and dry your feet well. When you shower, soap your feet and wash with warm water, and fully dry them, even between the toes. Moisture trapped between the toes can be harmful. Do not soak your feet, as excessive moisture can cause skin breakdown.

4. Wear shoes that fit well; ask your doctor about prescribing custom-fit roomy and comfortable diabetic shoes. Work with an orthotist who can take a mold of your feet and create special inserts. Keep your foot cushioned with soft socks; you need proper padding.

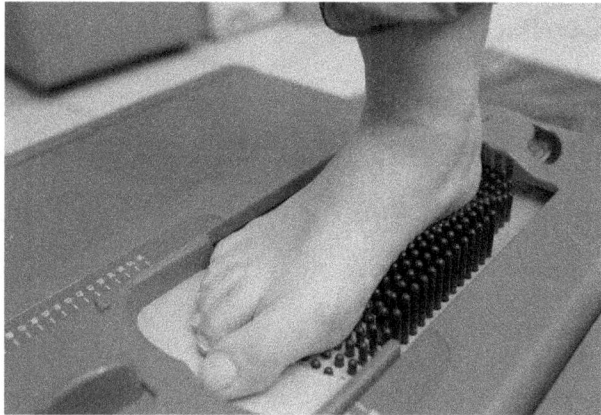

Foot scanning device for customized shoe inserts

5. Do not trim your toenails. See a podiatrist, a doctor who specializes in foot care. He or she will expertly trim your toenails to prevent you from cutting yourself and can trim your calluses to prevent pressure-related ulcers. You may be able to manage your calluses with a gentle filing device, pumice stone, and urea cream.

6. Use lotions or creams to keep skin from drying or cracking.

7. Avoid nail salons.

8. Two important things you can do to minimize the risks of neuropathy and vascular disease are to quit smoking (and avoid second-hand smoke) and get plenty of sunlight and exercise.

9. If you have neuropathy, protect your extremities (especially your feet) from temperature extremes. It is important to avoid burns and frostbite. Check water temperatures before immersing your feet and use care while cooking. Protect extremities during near or below freezing temperatures. Do not walk barefoot!

CONCLUSION

If you have diabetes and injure your foot or leg, do not try to take care of it at home. Put some antibiotic ointment, calendula ointment, or medical honey on it and see your doctor as soon as possible. If it does not heal quickly, then do everything possible to be seen at a wound center. The clock may be ticking.

References and Recommended Reading

1. Ruben, Bruce. "Osteomyelitis: What Is It and How Is It Treated?" *Woundsource.com*. Woundsource.com, 3 Mar. 2014. Web. 11 June 2017.

2. McKenzie et.al. "A Novel Intervention Including Individualized Nutritional Recommendations Reduces Hemoglobin A1c Level, Medication Use, and Weight in Type 2 Diabetes." JMIR Diabetes. 2017;2(1):e5

CHAPTER 4

Failures of the Medical System

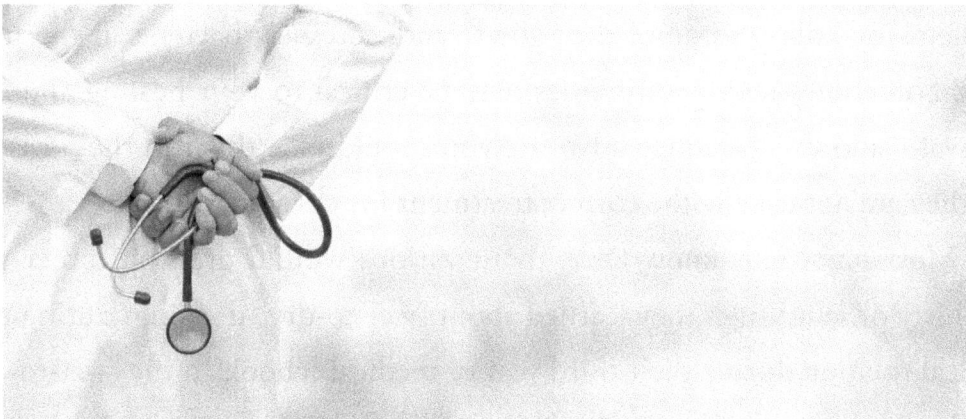

If you have a chronic wound and have sought help from your primary doctor, an urgent care clinic, the ER, or even have been hospitalized, you may not have gotten the kind of care that you need to heal your wound (if you are reading this book, it is likely). We have watched many patients struggle to get wound care they need—here's why.

MOST DOCTORS DO NOT KNOW HOW TO
TAKE CARE OF YOUR WOUND!

The majority of internists, family physicians, and emergency physicians have either little or no training in how to care for chronic wounds. Patients have told us their doctors have said "just cover it up" (so you or I do not have to look at it or think about it) or "let it air out and heal with a scab," or "it will never heal, so just get used to it," or "it looks infected, so I'll give you another prescription for antibiotics" or even worse "just put Betadine on it." (Betadine is excellent at killing not only bacteria but also the cells that help heal wounds.)

Most doctors prescribe antibiotics for nearly all wounds because they do not know what else to do, and sometimes antibiotics help. Some studies have shown patients are happier when they leave their doctors office with a prescription. Most of these antibiotic prescriptions are unnecessary and contribute to the worldwide problem of antibiotic resistance and can lead to substantial problems by killing some of the "good" and necessary bacteria in the intestines. Sometimes taking antibiotics may be critical to your healing and even survival—and we absolutely advocate you should take them in those cases—but they are not usually the correct treatment for chronic wounds.

Most physicians know little about various wound dressings other than the thirty or so minutes they learned about "wet-to-dry" dressings during their surgical rotation during their third year of medical school. In the "wet-to-dry" dressing, moistened gauze is placed into a wound and then covered with dry gauze. Eventually the moisture is wicked away by the dry gauze and then the whole dressing is removed. The now dried-out gauze sticks to the top layer of the (trying to heal) wound. This is like pulling a Band-Aid off and having the scab come with it (ouch!). Although reasonable for some wounds (usually fresh postoperative wounds), sometimes this technique pulls vital healing tissue off and causes more damage.

Surgeons do have experience and training to deal with wounds, either those they inflict or those that are referred to them. Most surgeons are extremely busy doing what they do best (operating) and thus do not have the time, energy, or interest to take on the care of chronic wounds—and they are not always up to date on the latest techniques as wound care has become a very specialized field. Orthopedic surgeons often view taking care of a chronic wound as a less-than-glamorous endeavor (compared to fixing broken bones,

replacing joints, doing arthroscopy, etc.), and since they are fairly adept at amputations, this is often the route they recommend.

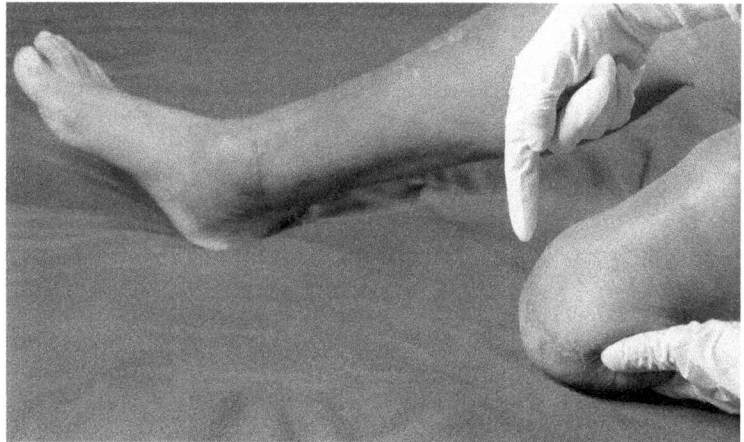

The sad cycle that occurs (and we have been part of it and have seen it innumerable times) is that primary care doctors do not really know what to do, so they prescribe antibiotics. Wounds do not improve, patients get frustrated, go to the ER, and the ER doctor prescribes more antibiotics and refers the patient back to their primary care physician. Eventually the patient is referred to or makes their way to a general or orthopedic surgeon and might end up with an amputation. Do not let this happen to you!

WHY THE HOSPITAL MAY BE THE WRONG PLACE FOR YOUR WOUND

You might be surprised to learn that even hospitalized patients do not receive optimal care for chronic and serious wounds. Although hospitals are the right place to receive care for many medical problems, healing chronic wounds is not one of them. It may seem incredible, but wounds often worsen while hospitalized.

Most hospitals specialize in treating acute (short-term and usually severe) medical problems. Hospitals are under tremendous pressure to reduce the average number of days that patients spend in the hospital because they are usually paid a fixed amount for the visit based on the diagnosis, not by how many days the patient stays in the hospital.

If you are admitted to the hospital for your infected chronic wound, you will typically be treated with IV antibiotics for a few days. As soon as the infection starts to improve, the impetus is to switch you to an oral antibiotic and discharge you. In some cases, the hospital will even try to set you up to receive IV antibiotics at home so you can be discharged even while still needing IV antibiotics. Does this sound familiar?

In addition, the wound care done in hospitals is not done by physicians specializing in wound care but by the nursing staff. If you are fortunate, you will have a certified wound, ostomy, and continence nurse (CWOCN). They can be a tremendous resource, but they have limitations—they cannot debride (remove dead and non-viable tissue) wounds using surgical instruments, obtain deep tissue cultures, prescribe the correct antibiotics when necessary, and they do not have ability to order the tests needed to necessarily diagnose or treat the underlying reason for the wound.

Most do not possess the sophisticated medical training to diagnose the underlying cause of the patient's health problems that led them to having a non-healing wound. Tragically, a surgical consultation might be requested before the patient has had

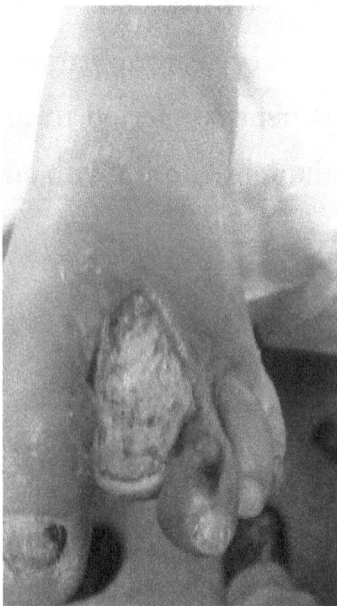

appropriate vascular testing. What do you think happens if you undergo a toe amputation with limited blood flow to your foot? Once the flap becomes necrotic, a BKA usually follows. This reflects the inconsistent and unreliable ability of physicians/surgeons/podiatrists not trained in wound care to recognize limb-threatening ischemia before debriding or amputating a toe.

In the next chapter, we will address where you *should* go to begin healing your wound.

References and Recommended Reading

1. "UK Doctors Create New Gel for Foot Ulcers." *Advancedtissue.com.* Advancedtissue.com, 10 Mar. 2017. Web. 11 June 2017.

2. Fife C, Carter M, et.al. "Cost to heal among 7900 patients at outpatient wound centers: data from the U.S. Wound Registry." *WOUNDS* 2011; 23 (3).

3. Reid R, Rabideau B, and Sood N. "Low-Value Health Care Services in a Commercially Insured Population," *JAMA Intern Med*; August 29, 2016.

CHAPTER 5

Wound Centers Offer Help

If you are fortunate enough to have a primary care physician who knows what they do not know about wound healing, you may be referred to a specialized wound care center. This can be tremendously helpful, although there are other alternative and often better ways to heal (as we will be discussing in the rest of the book).

WHAT HAPPENS AT A WOUND CENTER?

At our local wound center, 90 percent of compliant patients can be healed within twelve weeks with a median time of thirty days. Those are laudable healing rates but not easy to achieve. Here are the eight principles we follow:

1. Treating systemic conditions (especially vascular problems)

2. Identifying and eradicating infection

3. Improving diet and nutrition

4. Controlling edema (swelling) around the wound and of the extremity

5. Debridement and specialized dressings to eliminate biofilm and necrotic tissue

6. Moisture balance through correct dressing selection

7. Wound edge management

8. Protecting the wound from pressure, friction, and injury

We will discuss each of these principles in later chapters and how they apply to wound centers and what you can take from them to use at home to help heal your wounds.

At wound centers, the detailed intake process includes the patient's complete history of the wound, past medical and surgical history, physical examination, and evaluation of vascular status (which is critical to wound healing). Patients are also asked about lifestyle choices and receive brief counseling on nutrition and quitting smoking (if you want to heal, you *must* stop). Wound care physicians often consult with the patient's primary care physician to manage other relevant medical conditions and medications. Medications such as immunosuppressants, chemotherapeutics, corticosteroids, NSAIDs (aspirin, ibuprofen, and naproxen), and blood thinners interfere with wound healing, so alternatives are considered.

To assess blood flow (and healing potential) of the extremities, ankle-brachial indices (ABIs) and transcutaneous oxygen measurements (TCOMs), and vascular ultrasound or angiography studies are ordered. These help determine if a patient will benefit from a revascularization procedure such as vascular stenting or bypass surgery.

Sometimes other imaging studies (x-rays, CT [computerized tomography], MRI [magnetic resonance imaging], and ultrasound) are used to assess for infected pus pockets (abscesses), gas gangrene, or bone infections (osteomyelitis).

Wound care physicians follow patients weekly to evaluate progress and to debride new biofilm. Debridement is a surgical technique by which dead, diseased, or dying tissue, and a crusty or slimy layer known as biofilm is removed. As before, special attention is paid to the periwound skin and wound edges, from whence healing either stalls or proceeds.

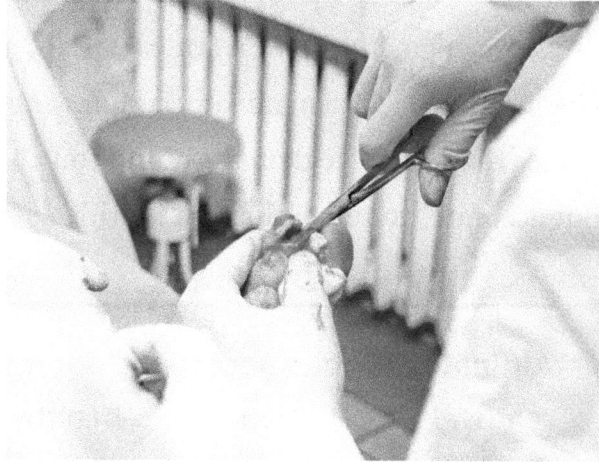

Specific deep tissue and sometimes bone cultures are taken when necessary. Cultures are reviewed to identify infections, and antibiotics are carefully tailored to the specific organisms, sometimes with the help of an infectious disease specialist. Deep wound infections and bone infections must be managed quickly and aggressively to prevent spread and facilitate healing. Necrotizing infections must immediately be identified and debrided to prevent sepsis and even death.

Diabetic ulcers require immediate intervention. Ulcers that do not achieve a 53 percent decrease in size by week four have only a 9 percent chance of healing over the next twelve weeks.

Pressure-relieving devices such as a wedge shoe, total contact cast, or AFO (ankle foot orthotic) are ordered. For more severe wounds, a knee scooter or wheelchair may be necessary.

Dressings are chosen based on specific wound characteristics and to optimize moisture balance. There are a multitude of options including specialized products such as collagenase, medical grade honey, silver impregnated dressings, alginates, topical antibacterials, absorptive foams, vacuum dressings ("wound vacs"), and many others. Dressing choices are far more varied, sophisticated, and effective than the ubiquitous "wet-to-dry" that most doctors order, but accurate wound evaluation is critical.

Alginate: Highly absorbent to manage heavy exudate, easy removal without damage to healthy granulation

Collagen: Provides a building block matrix for granulation and capillary growth, bio-absorbs into the wound bed, improves tensile strength of tissue

Foam: Absorbs large amounts of exudate, conforms easily to the wound, no pain at dressing changes

Hydrocolloid: Maintains a moist environment for wound healing, facilitates autolytic debridement of necrotic tissue, self-adhesive, adheres well to high friction areas, molds well to the wound

Hydrogel: Provides moisture to wound bed, gentle application and removal, reduces pain and scarring

These classes of dressings are available in a variety of shapes/sizes/thicknesses/forms.

Once the wound bed is appropriately prepared and treated, if it remains poorly healing after four weeks, insurance permitting (usually a lengthy paperwork process is required), specialized biological and tissue-based products are sometimes used. Many of these products are based on various types of stem cells such as human tissue and amniotic or umbilical cells.

Patients are continuously assessed for both potential benefit and insurance quali-fication for HBOT. Potential issues must be managed. For example, if a patient cannot clear their ears, pressure equalization (PE) tubes may be placed by an otolaryngolo-gist (ENT surgeon). Blood sugar must be carefully monitored in diabetic patients both before and during HBOT. Some patients require anti-anxiety medications for claustrophobia while in the chamber. Cardiac and pulmonary conditions (CHF, COPD, etc.) must be assessed prior to initiating treatment to determine if the risk outweighs the potential benefit of HBOT. A physician must be present to supervise all HBO treatments and deal with any issues or rare complications that arise.

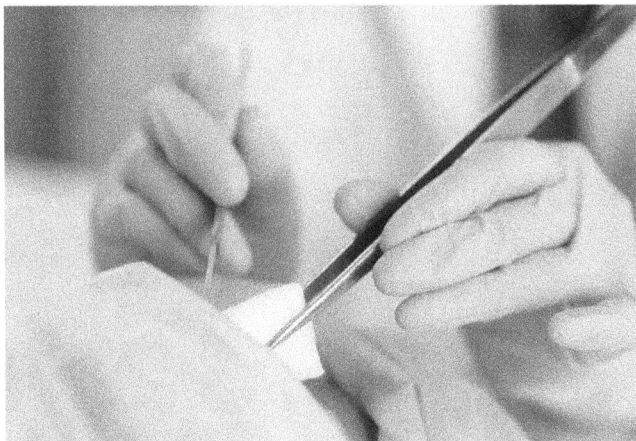

Case managers coordinate each patient's care and arrange for important needs including durable medical equipment (off-loading boots, crutches, wheelchairs, etc.), wound vacs (a special type of dressing and device that applies suction to help close wounds), dressing and bandaging supplies, home health visits, transportation, wound culture follow-up, IV line placement, outpatient intravenous antibiotic therapy, etc. There are numerous details to caring for complex and chronic wounds, and having dedicated staff to manage the process is critical for the best outcomes.

Many patients are accompanied to the wound center by family members or caregivers, and those caregivers are usually taught how to clean the wounds, change the dressings, and help with transfers and offloading, among other details.

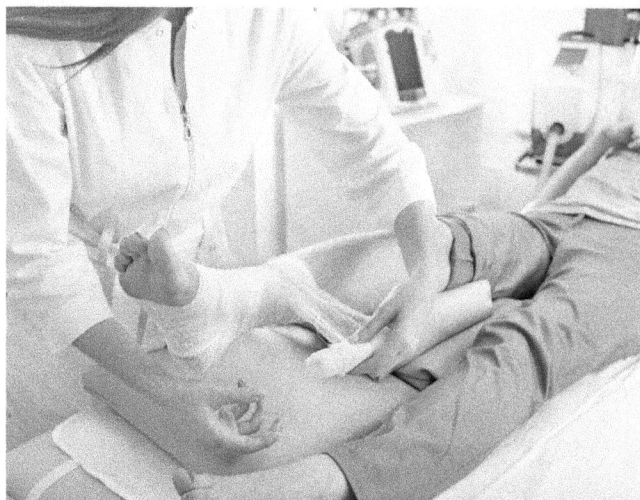

The physician group meets monthly to review challenging cases and share ideas and expertise.

This detailed, very resource-intensive approach, coupled with the expertise of physicians who have dedicated themselves to wound care, may produce excellent results and help heal very challenging wounds.

WHAT YOU CAN'T GET AT A WOUND CENTER!

Although wound care is a relatively new physician specialty, and the number of specialized wound centers has grown rapidly across the United States and worldwide, wound healing rates are not improving that much. Although we have the utmost respect for what happens in wound care centers nationwide, and we know they are the best option for many patients with chronic wounds, we will also offer some additional and sometimes better alternatives for helping you to heal. Application of the knowledge, techniques, and protocols we discuss in this book will help improve your health and vastly improve your chance of healing your wounds, even if you are already being taken care of at a wound center.

Most wound centers are reimbursed by billing insurance and are thus limited to providing treatments that are "approved" by mainstream medicine.

In the United States, the Centers for Medicare and Medicaid Services (CMS) has very strict criteria for paying for therapies, and most insurance companies follow CMS guidelines. For example, the rules for HBOT are constantly tightening (ask us how we know) to limit the use of this very effective but also expensive therapy (not nearly as expensive as the personal and financial consequences of a lost limb!).

Almost every wound benefits from HBOT, even if it does not meet CMS or insurance criteria for HBOT. So, if your insurance does not authorize it, another option is to find a "cash-based" HBOT center. These are typically found in larger metropolitan areas and charge "market rates" for HBOT. Because patients and their families are paying out-of-pocket, prices are usually more affordable than the inflated amounts that wound centers bill and get reimbursed from insurance or government entities.

These centers are typically started by entrepreneurial physicians (or chiropractors, naturopathic doctors, etc.) to treat "off-label" conditions. HBOT has been widely studied elsewhere in the world and benefits a wide variety of conditions including multiple sclerosis, head injury/concussion, stroke recovery, neurologic Lyme disease, severe infections, heart attack recovery, complex regional pain syndrome, burns, mitochondrial dysfunction, autism, and other developmental disorders. Such facilities rarely offer the specific wound expertise of true wound care centers, but they might allow you to get HBOT for your non-qualifying wound even while you are being seen at a wound center.

Another alternative is a home HBO chamber. Depending on your resources, they may be either rented or purchased. Be aware that they do not go nearly as "deep" as commercial grade chambers, but they provide some benefit.

Because of the insurance reimbursement model, wound care centers generally do not offer the alternative, natural, and experimental therapies that we discuss in the remainder of this volume. These include platelet rich plasma (PRP) therapy, light therapy, energy medicine techniques such as PEMF, ozone, natural topical products, chelation therapy, stem cell therapy, frequency specific microcurrent, and others.

Also, because wound care physicians are frequently under significant time pressure and narrowly focused on wounds, it is the rare one (still haven't met any others …) who will have the time, expertise, or inclination to dive deeply into a patient's hormonal milieu, nutritional status, chronobiology, toxic burdens, lifestyle factors, or many of the other issues we discuss in the pages that follow.

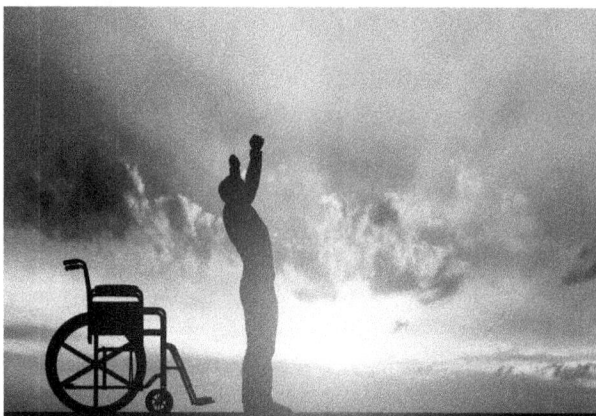

As you can imagine, these factors are what make all the difference in healing and reclaiming your health.

References and Recommended Reading

1. "4 Medications That Inhibit Wound Healing." *Advanced Tissue*. Advanced Tissue, 27 Jan. 2016. Web. 13 June 2017.

2. Sheehan P, et al. "A Percent change in wound area of diabetic foot ulcers over a 4-week period is a robust predictor of complete healing in a 12-week prospective trial." *Diabetes Care* 2003; 26 (6): 1879-1882.

CHAPTER 6

Heal Yourself, Heal Your Wound

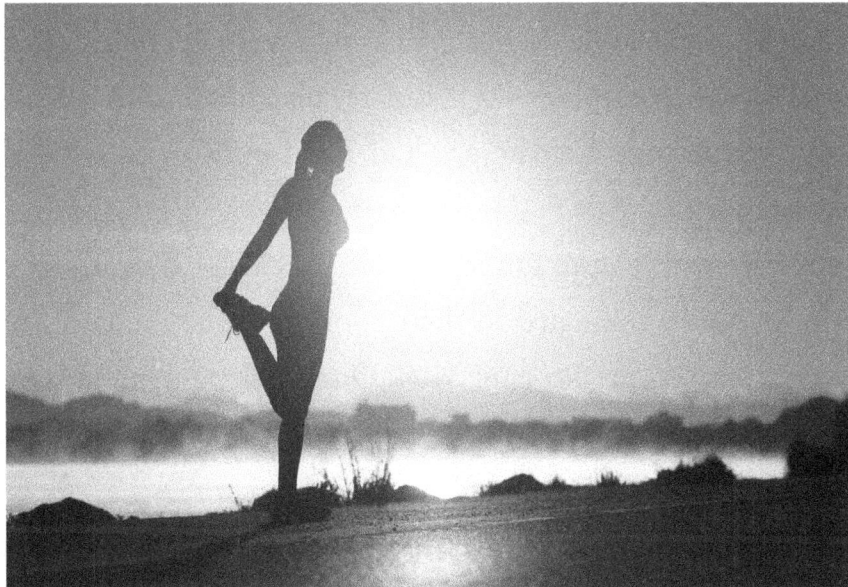

Chronic wounds are challenging. You are not likely to get the care you need in your doctor's office, the emergency department, or even a hospital. Our case reports, based on our real patients, illustrate how quickly and horribly things can go wrong. The multi-disciplinary teams at wound centers are a tremendous resource, but despite employing the latest wound management techniques, the most advanced dressings, and expensive industry-developed products, even wound centers fail some wounds. And frustratingly, about 65 percent of healed wounds recur within two years.

We know well the shortcomings of conventional wound centers (which are far better than most alternatives). Wound centers focus primarily on the wound, and this is emblematic of the problem with modern mainstream medicine. Many specialists focus only on the organ system they know best and do not consider the rest of the patient.

Our combined passions for wound care, alternative and regenerative medicine, along with interests in quantum biology and natural principles, have led us to a uniquely effective approach to healing. We believe it is critical to focus on the "whole patient" not just the "hole in the patient." We diagnose and treat underlying causative conditions, not the resultant non-healing wound.

Vibrantly healthy people do not get chronic wounds. Healthy bodies can heal given the right conditions. You can regain your health and heal your wounds by reconnecting with nature and tapping into your body's innate healing potential.

Reconnecting with nature sounds simple yet can be deceptively challenging. Most of us are so entangled in the trappings of the modern life that we may not even recognize our disconnection. Our bodies and brains have evolved over millions of years to be exquisitely attuned to the rhythms and frequencies of our planet. Our intelligence and ingenuity as a species has allowed us to create an artificial world that is convenient, comfortable, and enchanting, and yet operates detrimentally on our health.

Some of the following recommendations may sound far-fetched, off-the-wall, or unconventional to those who have yet to recognize the disconnection from nature that is at the heart of many modern diseases. We do not have the space to go into the science that supports each of them. Volumes have been written about each one, and more information can be found in the references. In addition to what is discussed in further chapters, here are important things to learn more about and do:

- Practice earthing. **Why:** The earth provides a (nearly) endless supply of negative electric charge (electrons), which counteracts the positive charges in our bodies associated with inflammation and electromagnetic fields (EMF). Our brains are exquisitely attuned to the natural electromagnetic frequency of the planet, known as the Schumann Resonance. **What you can do:** Spend as much time as possible (in an ocean or) in contact with the ground—preferably moist soil, grass, moist sand at a beach, or in contact with trees. Walk barefoot when you can and investigate special grounding footwear. If you are diabetic, you must approach being barefoot *very* carefully (i.e. do not walk, just set your feet in a safe place) to prevent new wounds. Consider purchasing grounding straps connected directly to earth. You might want to watch the documentary films *Grounded* and *Down to Earth* (out in fall 2017).

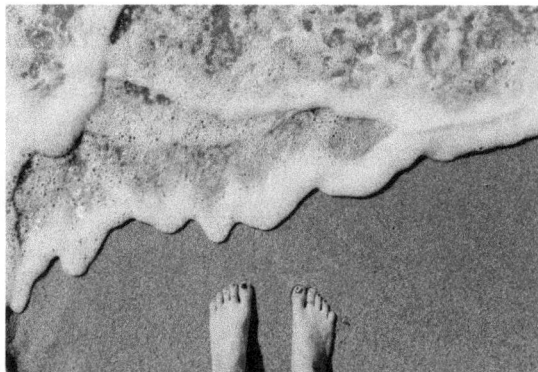

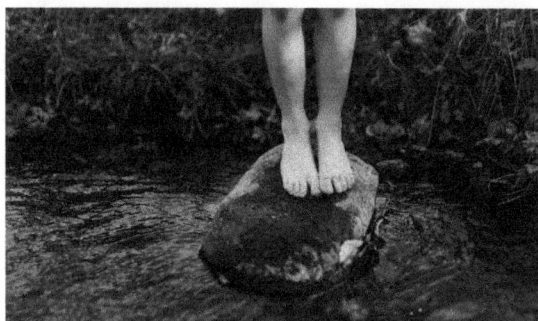

Although earthing/grounding is important, we do not recommend that diabetics walk barefoot. Do your earthing by picking a very safe spot (i.e. no rocks, twigs, thorns, sticks, temperature extremes, etc.) to place your bare feet on. Damp grass, sand, or a smooth rock or boulder is ideal. Sit with your feet there for a period. Do not move them around, wiggle them, or do anything that might cause trauma. Inspect them, clean them (get sand and dirt off), dry them, and then put your protective footwear back on.

"In simple terms, what Earthing does, is literally it squelches the fires of inflammation, and if inflammation is the source of all root illnesses, including Alzheimer's disease, cancer, heart disease, diabetes—I mean the list goes on and on—if you can impact inflammation and ... stop it, we're going to be healthier beings."

—Dr. Stephen Sinatra, cardiologist

- Avoid non-native electromagnetic fields (EMF). **Why:** The electrical nature of our bodies is well known, and every cell in our bodies and every mitochondrion in our cells depend on certain frequencies to operate correctly. The electromagnetic environment that is unseen around us has a *huge* impact on our health and vitality. New concerns arise nearly daily, but certain industries and economies based on these technologies are very much vested in suppressing these concerns. **What you can do:** Avoid Wi-Fi, cellular and mobile telephones, along with Bluetooth devices. Get rid of your microwave oven. If you live near power lines, cell towers,

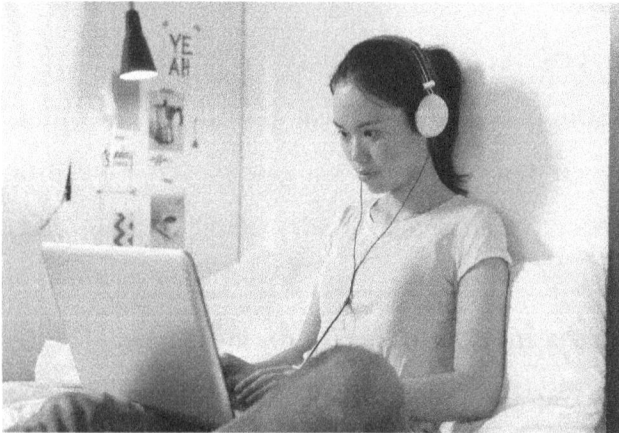

broadcasting towers, or in a crowded urban area, move. Mitigate "dirty electricity" in your home with filters and avoid, shield, or get rid of your "smart meter." We realize you may not be able to entirely avoid or eliminate these things, so learn ways to mitigate, including using "airplane mode" frequently and speaker mode on mobile devices, using shielded cables when possible for networks, turning off Wi-Fi when not absolutely necessary, etc. Distance from the source is critical—the power density of EMF decreases proportional to the square of the distance, so get as far away as you can.

Electromagnetic Spectrum

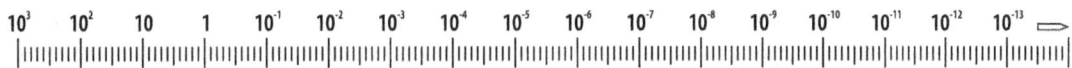
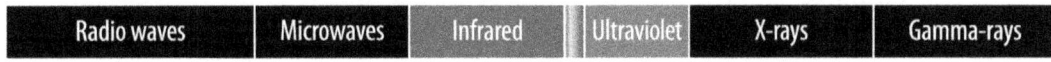
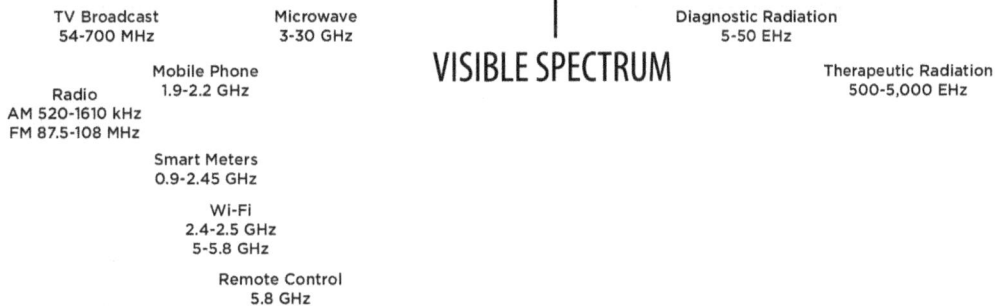
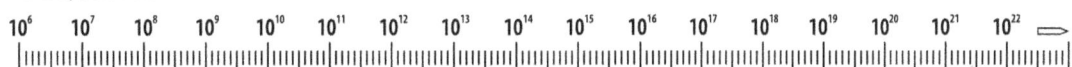
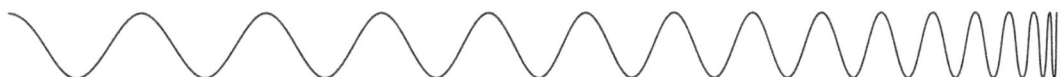

Courtesy of http://www.cancer.gov/about-cancer/causes-prevention/risk/radiation/electromagnetic-fields-fact-sheet.

- Drink lots of *good* water. **Why:** We are learning more about the critical role water plays in our bodies based on the implications of the recently described fourth phase of water (Exclusion Zone [EZ] water). Although water surrounds us (and makes up a large percentage of our bodies) and we take it for granted and think little of it, water is critical to cellular function and seems to have a huge role in cellular energy production and storage—the EZ allows it to act as a battery. Water has also capacity to store information by its structure. Hydration is critical (and by the way, EMF is dehydrating). **What you can do:** Drink lots of either spring water (preferably bottled in glass) taken from nearby springs or buy and use reverse-osmosis (RO) filtered drinking water. Avoid fluoridated or chlorinated water and seek water with the lowest Total Dissolved Solid (TDS) content for drinking. Learn about vortexing or other methods to structure your water. When your labs are tested, look at your BUN/creatinine ratio—it should be less than or equal to 7—this is an indicator of cellular hydration.

"Human cells run on light frequencies, not on calories, and only need ATP to unfold proteins to bind more EZ water. Then the cells can absorb more energy from the sun."

—Dr. Jack Kruse

- Embrace the cold. **Why:** As mammals, we have mechanisms to deal with temperature changes, and it is important to our biology that we feel the change of seasons. Unless you live (and eat) in an equatorial zone, biologically your need for cold correlates with the shorter light cycles of winter and different foods locally available. From the standpoint of physics, cold decreases the distance between proteins in your electron chain transport of your mitochondria and makes energy production more efficient. **What you can do:** Learn about the techniques of cold thermogenesis and start to apply them. Turn off or at least turn down the heat in your home. Start slow but work up to wearing less and less heavy outerwear when you are outside. Expose your body to the seasonal temperatures where you are. Sleep with fewer (no) covers. Use whole body cryotherapy if available near you (different mechanism but same general direction).

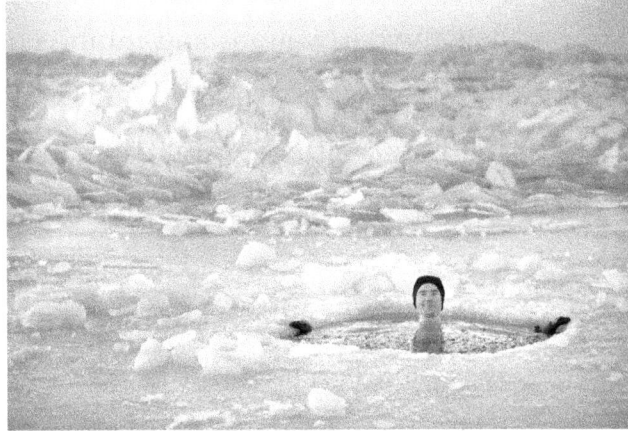

"Extreme" Cold Thermogenesis in the arctic

- Avoid environmental toxins. **Why:** This is a huge category to cover in a few sentences. Heavy metals (lead, cadmium, mercury, etc.) and aluminum can disrupt cellular function. Many pesticides (glyphosate, for example) and herbicides have been linked to neurodegeneration. Plasticizers (bisphenol A [BPA], phthalates, etc.) are endocrine disruptors (they usually mimic estrogen) and subtly change hormone levels, which can lead to significant problems. **What you can do:** Educate yourself. Buy and eat organic foods. Avoid non-stick cookware (use enameled, cast iron, or stainless steel). Use ceramic tableware rather than plastics. Avoid consuming processed or canned foods—fresh or frozen are best. Research vaccines that contain metal preservatives. Avoid herbicides and pesticides around your home. Move if you have significant exposures.

- If you smoke … quit! **Why:** Smoking is terrible for your health (you know that) and we are not going to rehash all the details here. It destroys your lungs and exposes you to literally hundreds of carcinogens, toxins, and noxious substances. From a wound healing perspective, the peripheral vasoconstriction it causes decreases blood flow to your wounds and inhibits healing. **What you can do:** There are volumes written and many programs to help you stop smoking, and now pharmaceutical companies have come up with a variety of (expensive) products that may help. Our recommendation is to freely use nicotine gums and lozenges (and even patches) to help wean yourself off smoking, but then wean yourself off the nicotine as soon as possible because nicotine is a vasoconstrictor. Combine the nicotine replacement therapies with lots and lots of good water and sunlight.

The next few chapters will discuss important topics including chronobiology, nutrition, hormones, supplements, and other ways to help create the ideal state for your body to heal. After that, we will get into specifics about how you should care for your wound. We will cover many topics including cleansing, dressings, and topical agents.

Finally, we will discuss some of the advanced and alternative techniques that are so effective for wounds. Some of these you can do on your own, but some will require you to partner with an appropriate practitioner, usually a physician. The holistic wound care program we have developed uses many of these techniques, carefully chosen for the specifics of the patient and the wound, to give our patients the best chance of success.

You are about to start a journey down the path to healing. Our mission is to illuminate the stepping-stones on that path. Touching each of those stones will provide a synergistic effect to heal you, as they have so many others.

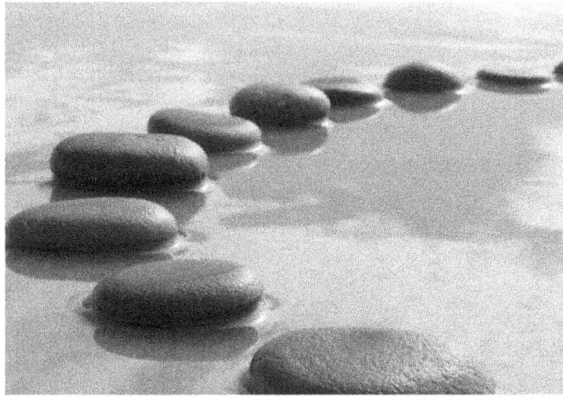

References and Recommended Reading

1. Ober, Clinton, Stephen T. Sinatra, and Martin Zucker. *Earthing: The Most Important Health Discovery Ever?* Sydney, N.S.W.: Read How You Want, 2014. Print.

2. Gittleman, Ann Louise. *Zapped: Why Your Cell Phone Shouldn't Be Your Alarm Clock and 1,268 Ways to Outsmart the Hazards of Electronic Pollution.* New York: HarperOne, 2011. Print.

3. Pollack, Gerald H. *The Fourth Phase of Water: Beyond Solid, Liquid, and Vapor.* Seattle: Ebner & Sons, 2013. Print.

4. Kruse, Jack. *Epi-paleo Rx: The Prescription for Disease Reversal and Optimal Health.* United States: Optimized Life PLC, 2013. Print.

5. Hof, Wim, Justin Rosales, and Brooke Robinson. *Becoming the Iceman: Pushing Past Perceived Limits.* Minneapolis: Mill City, 2012. Print.

CHAPTER 7

Timing is Everything:
An Introduction to
Circadian Biology

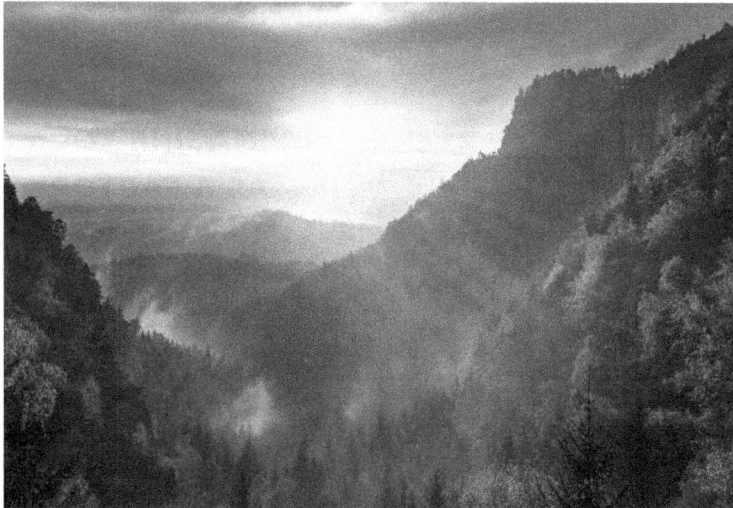

Very few people realize the importance of circadian biology to our lives (physicians included). Light (and darkness, and thus day and night) is fundamental to nearly everything about our biology. Every living thing on our planet

67

depends on the light of the sun. The energy carried from the sun to the earth by rays of light allows plants to grow and multiply, which feed animals, which ultimately allow human beings to live. Every living cell depends on sunlight in some way. Surprisingly, modern medicine has nearly completely ignored the importance of light to our biology.

We are evolved to distinguish between the light of day and the darkness of night and the important transitions between them. During the day, we gain energy from the food (and the sun), and, of course, all our food contains energy ultimately derived from the sun. At night, we depend on the absence of light for many important processes to take place. This is critical for optimal health, and unfortunately, many conveniences of modern life have given us the ability to completely ignore the natural rhythms of day and night, and this leads to disease and rapid aging.

A whole new field studying how our cells, hormones, and organ systems interact with the light and time of day has been developing. Scientists are now learning how critically important this timing is in our bodies. The study of this field is known as circadian biology or chronobiology.

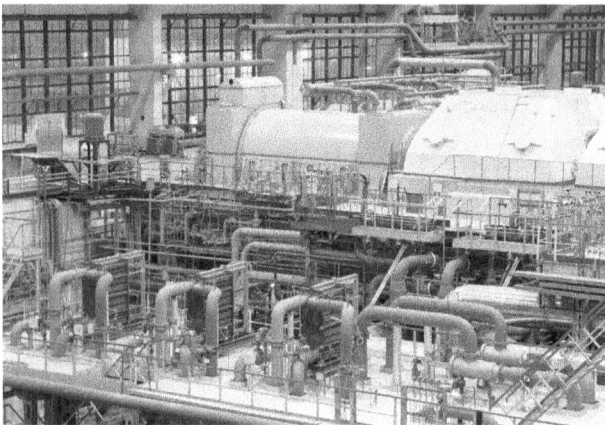

IMAGINE YOUR BODY AS A FACTORY

Your body is like an incredibly complicated factory with over one hundred thousand biological and biochemical reactions going on every second. Imagine the most complicated factory you can, producing many thousands of products, with thousands of assembly lines, hundreds of receiving docks where goods are processed and fed into the factory, and hundreds of shipping docks where products are loaded and shipped.

Many of the necessary raw materials for products in the factory are the same for many processes and must be shuttled to different points in the factory and then placed on assembly lines. Many outputs of certain assembly lines must be shuffled off to other assembly lines to provide materials to create other products. In the end, the factory must properly identify, label, organize, and ship hundreds of thousands of things to the right place at the right time.

In such an amazing factory, timing is critical. If everything is working perfectly, materials will be arriving at the multiple receiving docks, processed in a timely fashion and shuffled to their intermediate points quickly and efficiently, run through the appropriate assembly line processes to feed into other assembly line processes, with final products eventually sent to the shipping docks for output. Imagine that there are hundreds of steps in these processes, all of which require the correct timing to have the factory run efficiently.

If one assembly line stops working, products start backing up. This impairs the creation of products that require the output of that assembly line. The entire factory and the capability of producing the desired end products are affected. Products may not ship for days, or the wrong products might get shipped.

It is a mind-bogglingly complex system, and yet each of us, in our bodies, has these things going on all the time. Now, imagine the importance of the timing of all the different processes in your body. It is the same as the factory. If the timing is off in even one place in your body, problems result. Metabolic processes will become backed up. Things will not happen in the order they are supposed to. Products needed from one biochemical reaction will not be available for the next reaction, and ultimately the end products, which are your health, vitality, and ability to heal, will be badly compromised.

If everything is working well in the factory, we call this state *health*. When timing is off and products are beginning to pile up in a chaotic way, that is called *inflammation*. This is a lack of health. Depending on how badly the timing is off in any given system, that may determine whether that organ system is diseased. Much of this has to do with the health of those tiny little energy production factories in your cells known as mitochondria.

If the mitochondria of your heart are not working correctly, you may end up with arrhythmias, coronary artery disease, cardiomyopathy (a weak, damaged or enlarged heart muscle), and ultimately heart failure. The next stop on that pathway is death. If brain mitochondria are dysfunctional, you will likely end up with a neurodegenerative disease such as Alzheimer's disease, Parkinson's disease, or multiple sclerosis. If the timing of insulin production and metabolism is off, you will have diabetes.

CHRONOBIOLOGY AT WORK

A complex series of hormonal reactions takes place every morning when you wake up and see the first morning sunlight through your eyes. It starts certain chemical reactions, stops certain chemical reactions, changes the conformations of certain proteins and molecules, and effectively sets these critically important timing clocks that help synchronize every cell in the body.

For example, an important hormone called cortisol, also known as "the stress hormone," starts to rise a few hours before you awaken. It is your rising cortisol level that helps wake you up. It brings you back to consciousness from sleep.

Seeing the sun first thing in the morning is what tells your body that it is time to stop producing cortisol and start producing other hormones that you need throughout the course of the day. These are the hormones that allow you to eat, digest food, secrete digestive enzymes, and move about. This also includes your sex steroid hormones. In men, the predominant one is testosterone, and in women of childbearing age, this includes estrogen and progesterone. There are myriad other important events that this light signal synchronizes.

WHAT IS A HORMONE?

Hormones are chemical messengers in your body. The body has a multitude of ways of sending signals back and forth and creating and synchronizing activities. Signals can be sent via nerves, which are like cables or wires. Nerves go to one or more discrete places but cannot impact every cell in your body. Hormones are chemicals that, even present in small amounts, for example, picograms (which is one trillionth of a gram) per milliliter, have major effects on the body by binding to receptors on cell surfaces all over the body.

Examples of hormones include cortisol, insulin, human growth hormone, testosterone, estrogen, progesterone, melatonin, oxytocin, thyroid hormone, and vitamin D. Realize that the symphony of all your hormones working correctly together, in the correct amounts, at the correct times, provides critical information to keep your body as healthy as possible. When your hormones are disordered or not working correctly, you are unhealthy.

Throughout the day, the light from the sun changes. Sunlight that you see is composed of thousands of different wavelengths and frequencies of light. It has one specific composition (spectrum) in the morning, another in the afternoon, and another in the evening. It turns out that our bodies are exquisitely sensitized to the specific spectrum of sunlight that falls upon them (or does not when the sun is down), and this is in fact what sets our circadian clocks and keeps everything in that complex factory in our body running correctly.

As the sun goes down, another critical sequence occurs. During the day, the ultraviolet light from the sun falling on your retina (the back of your eye—essentially a part of your brain) helps regenerate ocular melatonin. As darkness falls, ocular melatonin signals the pineal gland in the brain, which produces pineal melatonin. Pineal melatonin eventually makes its way to the pituitary gland. Usually around 2:00 a.m., after you have been asleep for several hours and melatonin has been produced for several hours, there has been enough melatonin sensed by your pituitary gland to release a pulse of human growth hormone (HGH).

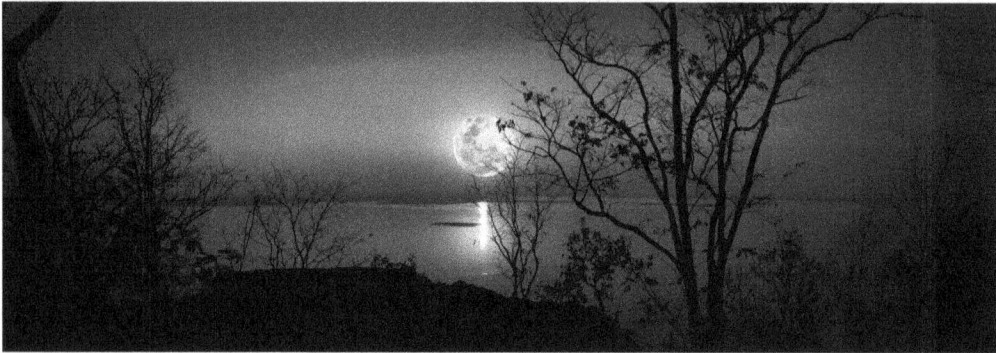

Some Hollywood stars and professional athletes have used HGH to enhance their looks, youthfulness, or athletic ability. It affects nearly every tissue in your body. Children without adequate HGH are very short, and in the United States, one of the only accepted uses for human growth hormone is to treat short statured children so they may attain a normal adult height. Once we attain our adult size and height, human growth hormone works differently on our body. It stimulates cellular repair (think wound repair). It helps keep your tissues young and repairs the damage done during the day while you sleep.

Imagine what happens to your body, the complicated factory, when timing is off. For example, if you stay up all night, you do not have any HGH for that night. If you do that every night, you will age more quickly as the damage you accumulate during the day will never be repaired (night shift workers beware). The primary purpose of sleep is to repair the damage during the day, and most people do not respect how important sleep is to their health.

In an age where there is entertainment (the Internet) and food available twenty-four hours a day, it is very easy to forget how important sleep is. We minimize the importance of it as we work on just one more project, try to meet just one more deadline, try to spend more time socializing with our friends, or play on social media or in front of the TV instead of going to bed.

Your body is not designed to eat at night. If you consume foods, particularly foods containing carbohydrates, either simple or complex, after your melatonin starts to be secreted, melatonin secretion stops, insulin secretion continues, and HGH is unable to bind to its receptors (insulin competes for binding). It may not be an issue occasionally, but if you habitually eat after dark, your sleep and repair processes will suffer. Your cells will never see the important stimulating pulse of HGH that helps them repair themselves, and your health will suffer and you will age more quickly.

LIGHT AND TYPE 2 DIABETES

These things are interrelated in more ways than you can imagine. It is the absence of light at night that turns off insulin secretion. Type 2 diabetes (T2D) is a disease of "insulin resistance." When you constantly have high insulin levels, eventually your cells become resistant to its effects. High circulating insulin levels have been proven to be very bad for your health, and one of the ways doctors check for early diabetes is to see what your insulin levels are. If they are high, you are most certainly headed toward

becoming diabetic. In T2D, your cells are ignoring all the insulin that your pancreas secretes.

Many of our patients tell us they are "insulin-dependent" diabetics. Most of these patients have T2D that is characterized by resistance to insulin, not the inability of the body to produce insulin. If you are a type 2 diabetic who must use insulin, your insulin receptors have been down-regulated to the point where your pancreas is unable to produce enough insulin to get their attention. Or even worse, the pancreatic cells that produce insulin have just shut down, wore out, or turned off after working too hard for too long. This means that you must use exogenously administered insulin. Most of the drugs commonly used to treat T2D sensitize your cells to insulin. If they no longer work, and you now must give yourself insulin shots, you have quite an advanced disease state.

Light and circadian biology is critical to your health. The absence of light at night turns down insulin production—your pancreas has receptors for the sleep hormone melatonin that shut down insulin production when melatonin is high (as it is supposed to be at night). Your body expects to see HGH at night, not insulin. Insulin and HGH have a similar shape, and if insulin is present, HGH cannot bind to its receptors. In fact, the way we estimate a patient's HGH secretion is to measure insulin-like growth factor 1 (IGF-1), which is made in the liver proportional to the nighttime HGH pulse. Attempting to correctly time and measure the HGH pulse would be difficult since it typically occurs around 2:00 a.m.

So, if you are diabetic and you allow a lot of light to hit your eyes and your skin at night, you are doing yourself no favors. You are making your diabetes worse. The disordered and non-natural light environment in which we allow ourselves to live may be the cause of the explosion of diabetes now.

Sound a little far-fetched? Not if you realize that our skin is nearly as sensitive to light as our eyes. Different frequencies of light penetrate our skin to various depths. Skin is a photoreceptive organ, and studies have shown that specific frequencies of light on the skin at night caused a decrease in melatonin secretion. In one study, a flashlight shined behind the knee at night caused melatonin levels to drop. This means less HGH secretion and less repair of cellular damage while you sleep.

The most important takeaway from this chapter is how important the natural rhythms of day and night are to your body, and how important it is for you to protect and respect those. The primary frequencies of light that suppress melatonin secretion are in the blue part of the spectrum. This is particularly concerning, because most of the technological devices that have exploded in popularity over the last ten years have LED (light emitting diode) screens that tend to emit a predominance of the blue component of light.

Most television sets, computer monitors, tablet computers, video games, and smart phones have a tremendous amount of light in the blue part of the spectrum. Fluorescent lights, including now-mandated compact fluorescent lights, and many LED lights have huge spikes in the blue part of the spectrum. The blue light from these devices essentially breaks down and destroys docosahexaenoic acid (DHA—a critical omega-3 fatty acid, the highest concentration of which is in the retina).

In addition to actual retinal damage (there is concern about an upcoming epidemic of blindness), blue light shuts off nighttime melatonin secretion. Does it make sense to you that perhaps all our technological devices, all our nighttime artificial lighting, and our twenty-four-hour lifestyles are keeping our insulin turned on all day and all night? Could this be contributing to the rise in diabetes? Absolutely.

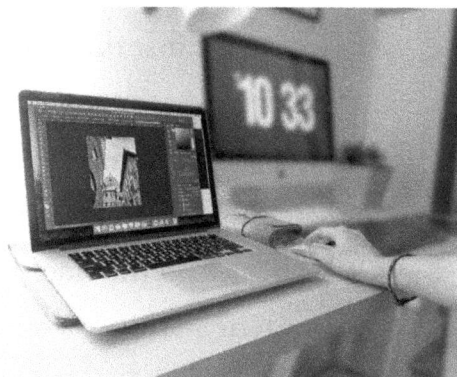

Unquestionably, high carbohydrate diets (especially after the sun goes down) also play a role in T2D. Too much dietary sugar, starch, high fructose corn syrup (soda), etc., certainly also contribute to diabetes. But the untold story, and what is not understood well yet by most of medicine, is how important the effect of artificial lighting, particularly light in the blue part of the spectrum at the wrong time of day is in creating diabetes.

Could this explain the fact that 55 percent of the population of California now has either diabetes or prediabetes? Could this explain the fact that children as young as three years old are now developing type 2 diabetes? Could this account for the fact that one-fifth of all new type 2 diabetes cases are diagnosed in teenagers, whereas this was unheard of twenty years ago? Absolutely.

WHAT YOU CAN DO

So what can you do about all of this? How can you protect yourself? What practical steps can you take to help heal yourself and respect your circadian rhythms?

Here is a list of things that you should think hard about, pay attention to, and may want to consider further research on. Just going through the details behind each one of these might well be enough to fill entire chapters. This is just a list of actions, from dawn until dusk, that will absolutely help improve your health.

- Go outside first thing in the morning and get sun, without any lenses (either glasses or contact lenses) on your eyes. The longer, the better. Eat breakfast, drink your coffee, read the news, or just enjoy the start of the day. Do not stare directly at the sun, look fifteen to twenty degrees off to the side. It is very important to get that sunlight onto your retina. This sets critical timing and starts the synthesis of ocular melatonin.

- Spend as much time outside in daytime sun as you can. If you have adequate nutritional intake of DHA, your body can harness energy from the sun (and you will not sunburn). You will have to build up to it, but you should expose as much skin as possible, and expose your wounds to sunlight. For centuries (before pharmaceutical companies…), ultraviolet light was used to cure many diseases, including tuberculosis, chronic wounds, depression, and others. Contrary to what modern medicine would have you believe, the sun is not your enemy. Studies have shown that people who regularly sunbathe live longer and healthier lives with less depression, cardiovascular disease, and cancer.

- Use as little sunscreen as possible, none is best. Sunscreen is a profitable modern product that ignores our biological need for sunlight on our skin. Of course, too much midday sun can cause a burn if you are not prepared for it. With time (it may take months or years) and proper nutrition, you will build a "sun callus" that will allow you to spend progressively more time in the sun. Most of us spend almost all our time indoors, and that is ultimately unhealthy. Being outside during the day helps keep your circadian rhythms synchronized and allows you to capture light and energy from the sun.

- Eat only during hours when there is still sunlight. Do not skip breakfast (unless you are fasting). Multiple studies have proven the importance of breakfast. When you wake up, the hormones in your gut have prepared you to receive and digest food. Do not disappoint them. Eat your larger meals earlier in the day and eat progressively smaller meals as the day goes on.

- Do not wear sunglasses when you are outside. If you wear contact lenses, take them out. If you wear glasses, take them off or look over the top of them frequently to get natural light in your eyes. Sunlight on your retina is critical to setting your circadian clocks. High-energy ultraviolet light recycles ocular melatonin. It is important that your brain senses the same light environment as your skin. With sunglasses, your brain and skin are getting two different messages. This discrepancy leads to chaos in our complex biochemical systems.

Biological Chaos = Inflammation = Poor Health = Aging

- As the sun goes down and darkness falls, turn out the lights. You have lighting in your home at night, but it should be of a kind that does not include frequencies in the blue part of the spectrum (red or amber—like a fire), as those decrease your melatonin production. Melatonin activates the HGH secretion, which heals you.

- If you must use a computer, tablet computer, or smartphone with a LED screen after dark, or watch TV after dark (you must?), wear blue-blocking glasses and cover as much skin as you can. There are applications available on the Internet that change the color of your smartphone or computer screen. Smartphone manufacturers have started to realize (or admit) the detrimental effects of blue light on health. In a recent operating system release, Apple introduced a feature called "Night Shift" which changes the color temperature of screens at night. Samsung is experimenting with different color temperatures for its LED screens. Absolutely use these. Some companies sell plastic blue-blocking filters to cover your screen. Great idea!

- If you need prescription glasses, we recommend blue-blocking lenses, especially if you spend a lot of time using computers or watching TV. BluTech lenses, Crizal Prevencia, Zeiss DuraVision BlueProtect, or others should be available at your local optometrist. If you do not need prescription glasses, and you spend a lot of time with screens, even during the day, you should get non-prescription blue-blocking lenses.

- If you wear prescription lenses, you can get a pair specially tinted that completely block blue light after dark. The lenses look orange or red. If you do not wear prescription glasses, you can cheaply purchase blue blocking glasses (try www.lowbluelights.com or Uvex Skypers) that completely block blue for after dark use. You will quickly get used to the color tint and notice an immediate improvement in your sleep—and consequent HGH secretion.

- Respect, protect, and treasure your sleep. Sleep is the most important factor in healing ourselves—it is when our bodies repair and regenerate themselves. The restorative HGH pulse is one of the critical mechanisms, but there are others.

- Create an optimal sleeping environment. Your bedroom should be entirely dark. All electronic devices should be removed. If you can possibly turn off the electricity to your sleeping area that would be ideal. If you have Wi-Fi or cordless phones in your home, turn them off at night, or better yet get rid of them. Although some people are more sensitive to the electromagnetic fields that these produce than others, these fields affect all of us, particularly during sleep.

- If you must get up at night, use an orange, amber, or red nightlight or flashlight. Do not turn on overhead lights as this will disrupt your melatonin flow and either cause difficulty getting back to sleep or diminish your quality of sleep.

CONCLUSION

Paying attention to circadian biology (chronobiology) is critical to your health. Your body is a complex system with thousands of reactions and processes that require precise and intricate timing. This timing is best set by the rhythms of our planet, including the sunrise, the sunset, the seasons, and other factors. Your return to health starts with paying close attention to these circadian rhythms and shaping your life around them. This may involve either shunning some modern conveniences or modifying the ways in which you live.

We know this sounds drastic and inconceivable. It may seem like too large a sacrifice, but if you want to heal your wound and reclaim your health and vitality, this is critical. You can drastically improve your life and your health. What is that worth to you?

References and Recommended Reading

1. Kruse, Jack. "Living an Optimized Life " Optimized Living PLC. Web. 13 June 2017.

2.   Bobby Hunt. "The Blue Light Diet - Change Your Light Change Your Life." *The Blue Light Diet - Change Your Light Change Your Life*. Stanford University. Web. 13 June 2017.

3. "Home – Chronobiology.com." *Chronobiology.com*. Web. 13 June 2017.

4. "LowBlueLights.com." *LowBlueLights.com*. Web. 13 June 2017.

5. 1940s UV Light Documentary: Ultraviolet Light Educational Film. https://www.youtube.com/watch?v=rn-Fbag_1v4.

CHAPTER 8

Eat Better to Heal Better

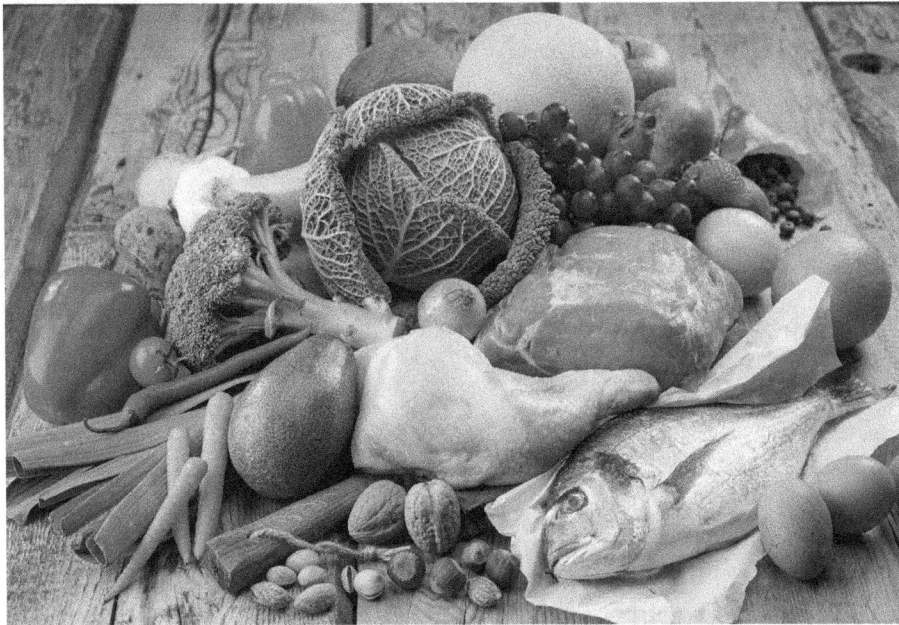

It takes a lot of energy to heal a wound. You must start with optimal nutrition and give your body the energy to heal itself. The old saying "you are what you eat" has a lot of validity when it comes to healing. Food provides the raw materials and the context that our body needs to heal itself. Estimates are that 40–60 percent of adults over sixty are clinically malnourished.

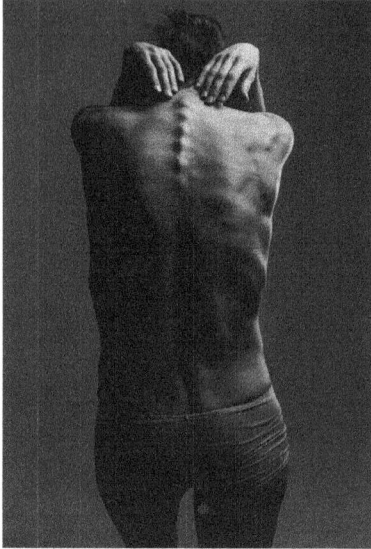

Malnutrition has three harmful effects on your wound: it prolongs the inflammatory phase, decreases the formation of collagen and blood vessels, and increases your risk for infection. Healing requires increased metabolism and thus energy demands. Without adequate nutritional intake, the body shifts to a "catabolic" state and breaks down muscle for necessary amino acid protein building blocks. This is ultimately harmful.

You can also be "overfed and undernourished." Nearly 9 percent of two- to five-year-olds are now obese. Since 1980, U.S. childhood obesity rates have tripled and the number of obese teens has quadrupled. Globally, 10-12 percent of adults are now obese.

In some measure caused by the rising obesity epidemic, now more than half of Americans struggle with chronic illness including chronic wounds, so it is critically important to pay attention to what you eat and to follow the advice given in this chapter.

One in five American deaths is associated with obesity.

—Dr. Joseph Mercola

The food you eat is a very powerful drug. It has tremendous influence over biochemical processes and controls such critical factors as inflammation, tissue repair, and even chronic pain. Some foods cause inflammation and low-grade immunologic reactions, which sabotage your ability to heal. Some foods contribute to "leaky gut" within your gastrointestinal tract. This allows toxins to seep across your intestinal barrier into your bloodstream. This causes chronic systemic inflammation, wrecks your health, and ultimately prevents healing.

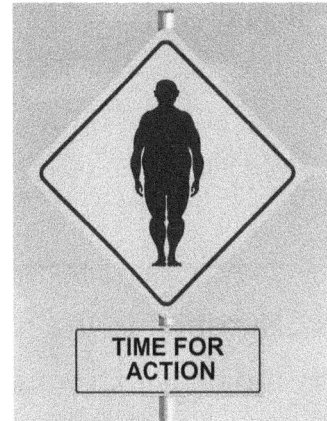

HEALTH OF YOUR GUT FLORA

Scientists and doctors are just starting to understand the importance of the billions of bacteria (of many different species) in our intestinal tracts. Collectively, they are called the "gut flora." Some estimates are that there are as many bacteria living inside of you as there are cells in your body. The proportions of different species of these bacteria matter. Some tend to promote health more than others, and certain compositions of gut flora lead to chronic diseases such as obesity and diabetes and may contribute to chronic inflammation and thus poor wound healing.

All disease begins in the gut.

—Hippocrates

Broad spectrum, powerful antibiotics disrupt the gut flora. Even though antibiotics are sometimes necessary for infection, well-meaning physicians who are either uninformed or just have tunnel vision, destroy your microbiome with the all-too-common practice of repeatedly prescribing for chronic wounds. In addition, the overuse of antibiotics is leading to bacterial resistance, diminishing their potential effectiveness for life-threatening infections where they are really needed.

EAT TO HEAL

Nutrition is the miracle the body performs when changing the molecular structure of food into living human tissue.

There are hundreds of books written on what you should eat. Most are very prescriptive "eat this, don't eat that, etc." (That is actually the title of a book.) Rather than replicate those, we will make a few specific dietary recommendations, and we absolutely recommend picking up any or all the books listed in the references for more details on the type of diet best for you.

If you want to heal your wounds and reverse many of your diseases, eat a moderate to high protein, low-glycemic index, low-carbohydrate, seafood-based, "Paleo"-type diet. It should be ketogenic in the winter and include more carbohydrates in the summer. If you are not familiar with this type of eating style, there are several excellent books including books by Dr. Jack Kruse, Robb Wolf, and Dr. Loren Cordain that can help introduce you to this type of eating. You may want to spend some time searching for more information on ketogenic diets on the Internet. Ketogenic diets are generally very high in healthy fat content (coconut oil, grass fed butter, ghee, avocados, olive oil, nuts, etc.). These type of diets have shown tremendous success at controlling and even helping reverse Type 2 Diabetes. Avoid modern processed foods. Shop around the periphery of most supermarkets.

Our bodies adapted and were designed to eat foods we could procure by hunting, fishing, or gathering. These include fish, shellfish, meats, vegetables, fruits (in season), and nuts. Food you should not eat include grains (wheat, corn, oats, rye, etc.), sugar, legumes (beans, including peanuts), and dairy products (although some people handle dairy better than others). Our bodies are also adapted to periods of fasting and lack of food, and intermittent fasting has actually been shown to be a powerful tool in reversing insulin resistance, facilitating weight loss and even potentially reversing diabetes. See Dr. Fung's books in the reference section for more details.

Eliminating (or at least substantially reducing) your consumption of those "non-ancestral" foods may help you to lose weight, decrease inflammation, and control or help reverse the symptoms of many diseases, such as diabetes, rheumatoid arthritis, lupus, fibromyalgia, thyroid problem, bowel problems, etc. You will feel better and more energetic.

Supermarkets, microwave ovens (do not use them), processed foods, foods in boxes, jars, cans, etc., are relatively recent (thirty to forty years old) innovations in human history. Despite industry sponsored, seemingly well-meaning (but tragically wrong) United States government guidelines on nutrition over that same time, there has been an explosion of diabetes, obesity, heart disease, brain disease, and auto-immune disease. Although food is certainly not the only explanation for this—circadian biology and light may be a bigger driver—food is an important thing to pay attention to as you try to regain your health.

We know that the thought of "never eating _____ again" (insert your favorite food—jelly donuts?) is daunting. Just commit to this style of eating for at least one month and see how you look and feel. You may decide that it just is not worth it to your health and sense of well-being to eat things that make you feel tired or sick, or perhaps you start eating them only occasionally, which is way better than all the time.

1. SEAFOOD

A seafood-based diet is recommended because of the omega-3 fatty acid, doco-sahexaenoic acid, also known as DHA. DHA is found in every cell (and cell membrane) in your body, and most of your brain is composed of it. DHA is essential to neurologic and cardiovascular health and critical for wound healing.

At the quantum biology level, DHA converts energy from incident light to cellular energy using the photoelectric effect. A detailed discussion is well beyond this book. DHA is best obtained from seafood. Eating food very low on the food chain will reduce concerns about toxins such as mercury. Other nutrients in the seafood will also help counteract some of the toxins. In order of best to worst, you should eat shellfish, crustaceans such as shrimp and crab and lobster, small fish such as sardines and anchovies, followed by larger cold-water fish such as salmon and halibut. Fresh-water fish (trout, bass, catfish, etc.) do not count as seafood.

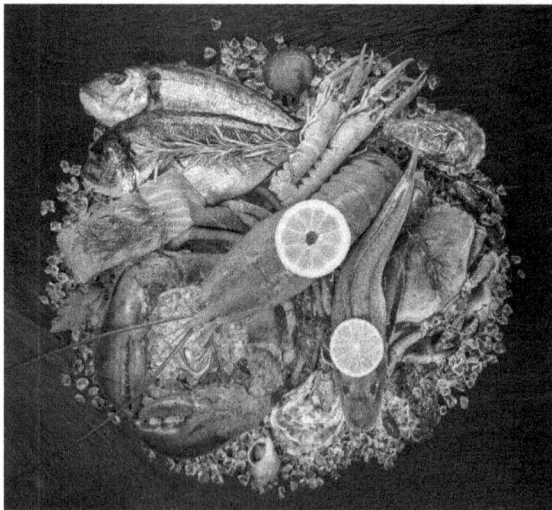

Seafood is one of the most nutrient dense foods on the planet, and in addition to DHA and other healthy omega-3 fats, it contains significant amounts of important trace minerals (such as zinc, selenium, etc.), vitamins, and anti-oxidants. Seafood is also high in protein and low in carbohydrates. Recent evidence shows that the human brain evolved largely due to diets rich in coastal shellfish and the DHA they provide, and a huge part of restoring your brain and thus body health is seafood consumption.

2. PROTEIN

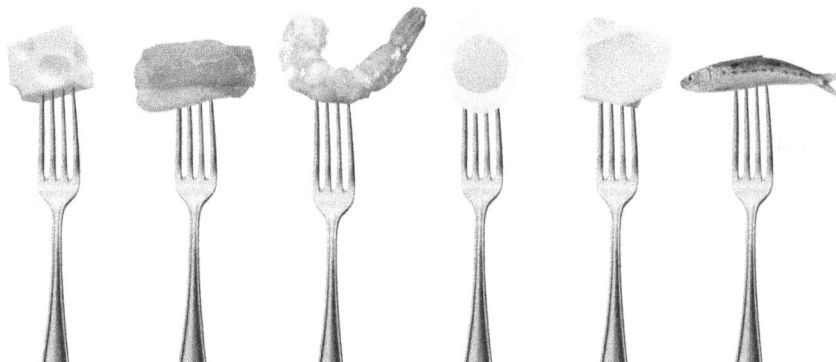

Adequate protein is critical to wound healing. Your skin, muscle, and connective tissue are largely built of proteins. Proteins are combinations of amino acids, and without adequate amino acids your body cannot rebuild missing or damaged tissue. Several studies have looked at the amount of protein necessary for optimal wound healing. Healing chronic wounds typically requires at least 1.5 grams of protein per kilogram of body mass per day (0.7 g/lb/day)—about a hundred grams of protein per day for most adults. If you are severely malnourished, have more than one wound, or greater than a stage 3 pressure ulcer, you should increase your protein intake to 2 g/kg/day. Although we do not specifically recommend you weigh and measure food, just remember that without adequate protein intake your wound will never heal, so focus on lots of protein-rich foods in your diet.

The best source of protein for those in need of healing is natural and unadulterated by hormones and antibiotics. A principle of the Paleo diet is to either eat *wild-caught* seafood or grass-fed meat. Although seafood is ideal, it is not always affordable or obtainable,

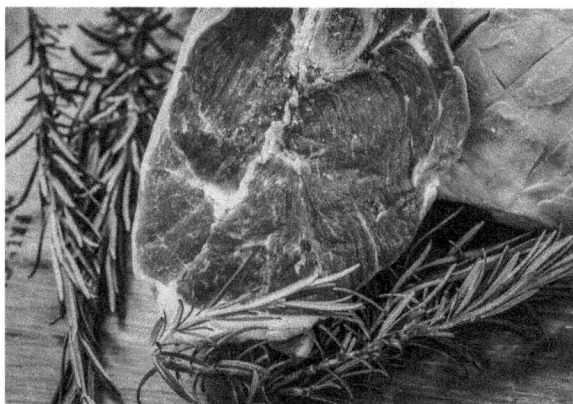

but grass-fed meat (or wild game) is better than most other sources. Grass-fed meat is so important because it contains fewer toxins, pesticides, antibiotics, and chemicals than conventional grain-fed beef. Grass-fed meat has a much higher DHA concentration than grain-fed meat. Although protein shakes and bars (which usually contain whey protein) can be used occasionally, they should not be staples of your diet. Study after study has shown that populations that live near a coastline with heavily seafood-based diets are the healthiest.

3. GRAINS

Grain has only been domesticated in the last ten thousand years or so. In fact, there is some data suggesting that tooth decay and obesity started to become prevalent when people settled down from being hunter-gatherers to the relative security of farming, raising, and eating grain. Many of our modern grains have been genetically modified, and most of you have probably read and heard about the epidemic of gluten sensitivity.

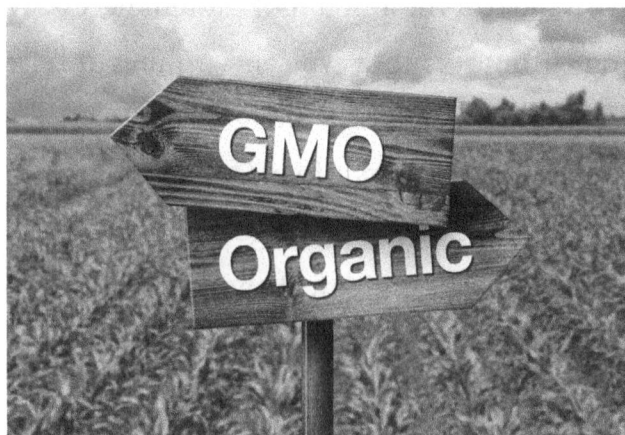

While not everyone is gluten sensitive, most are. Gluten and gliadin are proteins found in wheat and cause "leaky gut," which allows toxins found in your gut to seep across the gut membrane and cause inflammation. If you are sick enough to have a chronic wound, then you need to do everything you can to avoid this problem, and staying away from grains and gluten is an important component of this. In addition, most corn in the United States is genetically modified. Just stay away from grains of all types.

A low glycemic index diet focuses on not eating starchy or sugary foods that cause your blood sugar to skyrocket quickly. This will help you control your blood sugar, improve your blood lipid panel (cholesterol and triglycerides), and help you to lose weight.

4. VEGETABLES

Eat lots of them. Nutrition and health start in the soil. Fiber-rich vegetables not only provide valuable nutrients your body needs but also provide nutrition to the microbes in your gut, which feed on fiber. Eat vegetables grown in healthy soil, not factory-farmed vegetables grown in nutrient-poor soils. Ideally you will replace sugary foods and grains with a significant amount of vegetables. Stringy vegetables like artichokes, celery, and asparagus are high in inulin (not insulin) that feed gut bacteria.

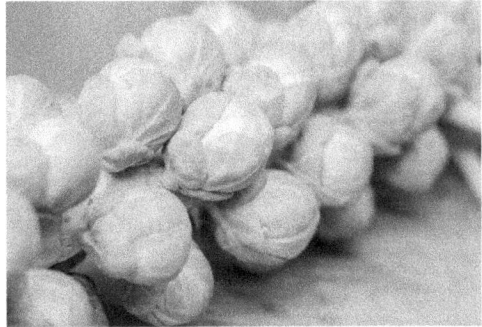

5. FRUIT

If you are diabetic or have any issues with blood sugar control, then you need to be very careful about fruit intake. Although fruit is generally healthy and contains lots of important vitamins, antioxidants, nutrients, and fiber, it also has a fair amount of sugar. The fruit you should focus on are berries as they have the lowest glycemic index, and always eat the fruit that is naturally in season in your area. In the winter, during low-light periods, you should avoid fruit altogether.

Buy organic produce. Many of the pesticides and herbicides (think Round-Up [glyphosate]) used in commercial farming are endocrine disruptors.

They either mimic or block the action of critical hormones within your body. Your body is an incredibly complex system, and changing hormone actions or blocking them leads to molecular chaos and inflammation and reduces your chance of healing.

If you cannot afford to buy everything organic, make sure to check the Environmental Working Group's website (www.ewg.org). They periodically test fruits and vegetables to determine which have the highest pesticide residues and publish a list called the "dirty dozen" which directs you to what twelve things you should buy organic.

References and Recommended Reading

1.   Kruse, Jack. *Epi-paleo Rx: The Prescription for Disease Reversal and Optimal Health*. United States: Optimized Life PLC, 2013. Print.

2.   Wolf, Robb. *PALEO SOLUTION: The Original Human Diet*. S.l.: TUTTLE, 2017. Print.

3.   Cordain, Loren. *The Paleo Diet: Lose Weight and Get Healthy by Eating the Food You Were Designed to Eat*. New York: Wiley, 2003. Print.

4.   Shetreat-Klein, Maya, and Rachel Holtzman. *The Dirt Cure: Growing Healthy Kids with Food Straight from Soil*. New York, NY: Atria, 2016. Print.

5.   Chutkan, Robynne. *The Microbiome Solution*. Sydney: Read How You Want, 2017. Print.

6.   *Overfed and Undernourished*. Dir. Troy Jones. *Https://www.facebook. com/overfedandundernourishedmovie/*. Gravitas Ventures. Web. 13 June 2017.

7.   "Eat Wild." *Eat Wild*. Web. 13 June 2017.

8. "Home." *The Weston A. Price Foundation*. WAPF. Web. 13 June 2017.

9. "EWG." *EWG*. Environmental Working Group. Web. 13 June 2017.

10. Mercola, Joseph. *Fat for Fuel: A Revolutionary Diet to Combat Cancer, Boost Brain Power, and Increase Your Energy*. Carlsbad, CA: Hay House, 2017. Print.

11. Fung, Jason. *The Obesity Code: Unlocking the Secrets of Weight Loss*. Greystone Books, 2016.

12. Fung, Jason, and Jimmy Moore. *The Complete Guide to Fasting: Heal Your Body through Intermittent, Alternate-day, and Extended Fasting*. N.p.: Victory Belt, 2016. Print.

CHAPTER 9

Optimize Your Hormones

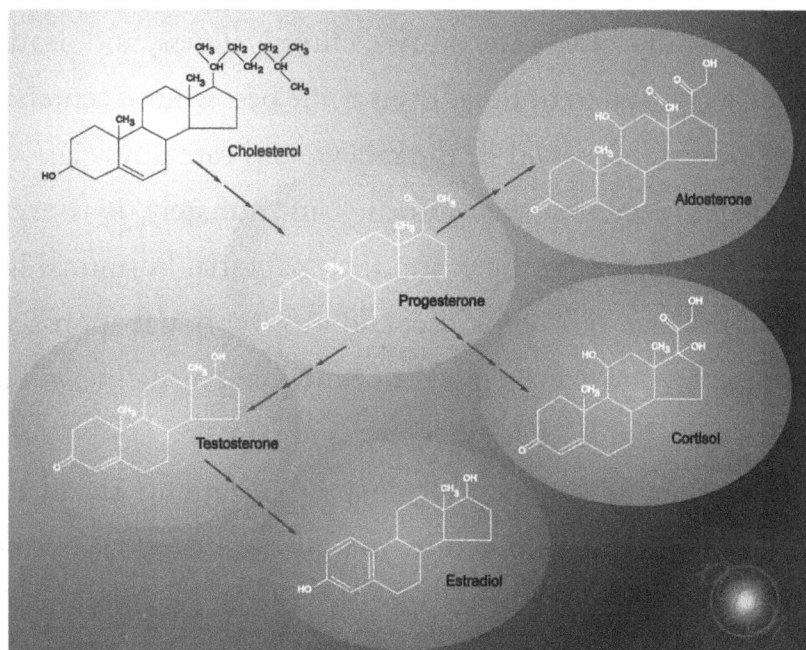

Hormones are important chemical messengers in your body that control numerous systems and bodily functions. They control protein synthesis and degradation, growth, tissue repair, mood, and body composition. They tell your body when it is time to wake up and go to sleep. They control hunger and thirst and signal your brain when you have had enough to eat. Hormones prepare you to face danger and stress, help you relax and unwind, control attraction, and facilitate reproductive behavior. They are the biochemical basis of human emotions, including love and attachment. And … they control the healing of your wound.

Hormones kick off the process of puberty and create the huge physiologic, psychological, and physical changes that turn us from children into men and women. With age, many hormone levels decline (exceptions to that are cortisol and insulin). Some of this decline is programmed into our bodies—i.e., in the fifth or sixth decades; women enter menopause and specific hormone levels decline. Many men now go through a similar process known as "andropause" as their testosterone levels decline. Biologically and evolutionarily, these changes signal the end of fertility and vitality and the long, slow (or worse, rapidly progressive) decline into disability, disease, chronic illness, and death.

Hormones are critical to healing. Even at the best wound centers, the focus of care is your wounds. It would be the rare wound care physician who would consider and treat your hormonal milieu. Unfortunately, it is even rare for many primary care doctors to check and treat potential hormonal issues. This is where the knowledge, skill, expertise, and interventional approach of those trained in anti-aging, age management, or functional medicine will be of *huge* benefit to you.

If you follow the advice in prior chapters regarding circadian biology, nutrition, and reconnecting with nature, you can optimize your hormone levels for your situation (it will take months though). If you are suffering with a non-healing wound and you are over thirty-five or so, your underlying problems make it likely that you will benefit from hormone treatment/replacement. This is where modern medicine can be helpful if you find the right doctor. Your body relies upon more than fifty known hormones, but we will focus on a few easily measured and treatable ones.

VITAMIN D

Vitamin D is misnamed. It is a hormone, not a vitamin. Vitamins are necessary cofactors in enzymatic biochemical reactions in your body, and they cannot be synthesized in your body—that is, we must get them from food. Vitamin D (also known as cholecalciferol) is a hormone made in your body by the action of ultraviolet light on cholesterol in your skin. You can obtain about 10 percent of what is needed from your diet, but the rest must come from your skin. *If you do not get enough sun—you will not have an optimal vitamin D level.*

Low vitamin D levels have been linked to a number of diseases, including various cancers, cardiovascular disease, osteoporosis, type 2 diabetes, chronic inflammation, age-related macular degeneration (the leading cause of blindness), and Alzheimer's disease, among others. Optimal vitamin D levels are estimated to decrease cancer risk by up to 60 percent for at least sixteen different types of cancer, including pancreatic, lung, ovarian, prostate, and skin cancers.

Of course, vitamin D levels are correlated with wound healing. For example, a 2012 study from Brazil on patients with venous leg ulcers showed those with higher vitamin D levels healed much faster.

Recently, many physicians have recognized that vitamin D deficiency is serious and very common; there is now a pandemic of vitamin D deficiency. Many recommend testing and oral supplementation because of a widespread (yet fallacious) belief that vitamin D deficiency is easily correctable by taking supplements.

Consider: An optimal vitamin D level is required for health. Our bodies manufacture vitamin D when exposed to sunlight. Thus, sunlight is necessary for optimal health (remember the transitive property of equality: if A=B and B=C, then A=C). Of course, vitamin D is not the only product of exposure to sunlight or the only reason we need sunlight; it is simply one marker of health that we have been able to correlate with sunlight exposure. Remember this: *Vitamin D from a pill does not carry the same quantum signal to your body that vitamin D created in your skin from exposure to UV light does. The sun brings great health; you should embrace it.*

Unfortunately, exposure to natural sunlight has been loudly denounced both by many physicians and by an industry eager to make huge profits selling products designed to protect people from the "harmful rays of the sun." Because of this we are seeing a correspondingly significant increase in cancer, cardiovascular disease, and a host of other ailments as the populace obediently tries to avoid the sun and slathers on sunscreen, covers up, and spends most of their days out of full-spectrum sunlight. The sun is the source of all energy on earth, and to think that our bodies have not optimally adapted to it (and are dependent on it) over millions of years is foolish.

Despite what you may hear from dermatologists, more recent studies have shown that sun exposure helps *prevent* skin cancer. Melanoma occurrence decreases with greater exposure to direct sunlight. For example, in a study published in the *European Journal of Cancer,* melanoma was more common in those who spent time indoors and in body parts not typically exposed to the sun. Another study showed that those who regularly sunbathe live longer. In the United States, skin cancer rates are highest in some of the states with the least sunlight (for example, Washington and Maine.)

We strongly recommend ample midday sunlight exposure on as much exposed skin as possible (yes, nude if you can—work up to it) as your main source of vitamin D. There are smartphone and computer applications that tell you when the best time to get maximal UVB exposure is (it is usually around noon, but the length of UVB availability will vary depending on your latitude and season). The strength of the sun's rays (measured by a concept called "quantum yield") will be less in heavily populated areas with lots of air pollution and competing electromagnetic waves (non-native EMF).

If you live in a climate where you cannot get adequate sun exposure (UV light) during the winter (or anytime), consider using tanning beds a few times a week (protect your eyes though). The benefits of optimizing vitamin D levels will outweigh the risks of the additional EMF.

While adequate sunlight is essential, sunburns are definitely miserable and can be harmful. If you are not accustomed to sunlight exposure, start with small amounts and work your way up to build your "sun callus" which takes time and effort. It is also critical to have a large amount of docosahexaenoic acid (DHA—the omega-3 fatty acid found in seafood) in your diet, and be well hydrated with good quality water. These measures help prevent burns.

Your goal is to get your vitamin D level into the optimal range: 70–100 nanograms/milliliter (ng/ml) as measured by most labs. Have it checked regularly and expect some normal variation with season depending on where you live. If you cannot get your vitamin D into an optimal range with sun exposure (change your lifestyle—you must!), we definitely recommend oral supplementation for a few months as you heal.

Most multivitamins have a paltry amount of vitamin D (200-400 International Units [IU]). That will not improve most people's vitamin D deficiency; the majority that we have tested have levels much less than 20 ng/ml. You may need anywhere from 5,000–25,000 IU per day. It is nearly impossible to become

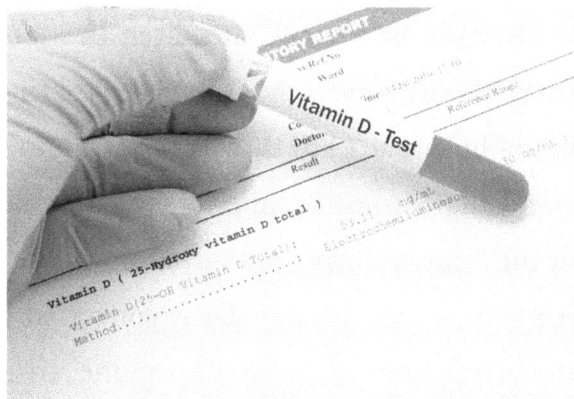

vitamin D toxic (levels greater than 150 ng/ml or a rising blood calcium level). Testing it periodically to follow the level is definitely important.

If your vitamin D level does not improve despite copious sunlight and/or aggressive supplementation, it is likely that your environment is the problem. This happens when there is significant electromagnetic pollution (nnEMF) because calcium is effluxed from your cells under these conditions. Because vitamin D increases calcium absorption in the gut, high extracellular calcium signals your body to decrease vitamin D levels. Systemic calcium levels are tightly controlled by the body, as the right concentration is critical to muscle (including cardiac muscle) activity.

Another potential issue that can cause your vitamin D level to be low is the mismatch created when your extremely photosensitive skin is exposed to sun but your eyes are not. Ditch the sunglasses (and the glasses and the contact lenses) and get some sun on your retina. Your brain must sense similar signals from your retina and your skin in order to maximize vitamin D levels.

THYROID HORMONE

A critically important and often overlooked hormone for wound healing is thyroid hormone. The pituitary gland (in your brain) produces thyroid stimulating hormone (TSH), which acts upon the thyroid gland, a butterfly-shaped gland that sits astride the trachea (in your neck). TSH stimulates production of the "storage form" of thyroid hormone called thyroxine (abbreviated T4 – it has four iodine atoms). T4 is converted by the removal of an iodine atom to the active form of thyroid hormone, tri-iodothyronine (T3). This conversion occurs in the bloodstream, the liver, the brain, and other "target tissues" of the body.

In addition to adequate iodine in your diet, a number of other trace elements and micronutrients such as selenium, zinc, iron, and many of the B vitamins are required for proper thyroid function. A nutrient rich diet with lots of seafood (and seaweed), grass-fed meats, and fresh vegetables provides the essential nutrients.

T3 controls your metabolic rate and the transcription of many genes, which affects wound healing. Those with hypothyroidism (low thyroid hormone levels) experience many symptoms including feeling cold, lack of energy, inability to lose weight, weight gain, thin/dry/brittle skin, loss of the outside portion of eyebrows, problems with hair falling out, depression, slow or foggy thinking, poor wound healing, and a variety of other problems.

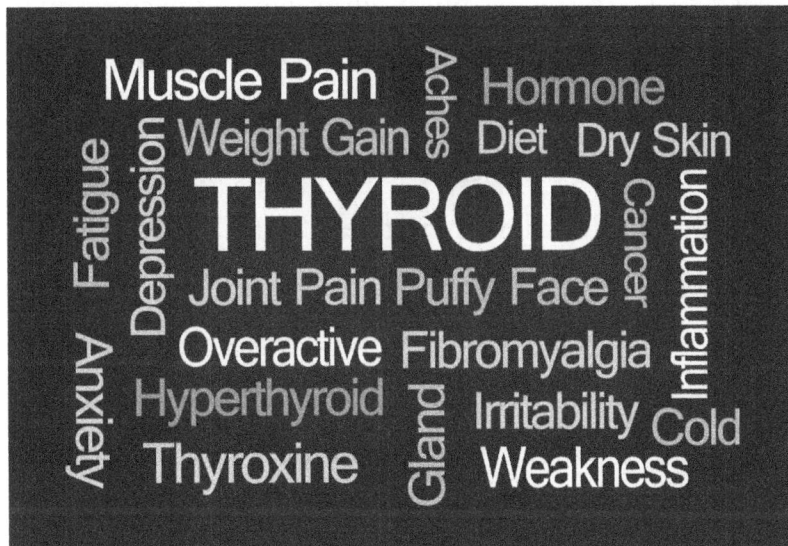

Unfortunately, many physicians only diagnose thyroid deficiency when the TSH level goes very high or at least when it goes above the so-called "normal range." When the brain senses low T3, it increases TSH to stimulate the production of more T4, hopefully to be converted to T3. However, the brain has different sensing mechanisms for appropriate T3 levels than many other tissues, so even if the brain senses an "appropriate" level of T3, various target organs in your body may not be getting enough T3 and you could continue to suffer from hypothyroid symptoms.

Anti-aging and functional medicine physicians often diagnose hypothyroidism by looking at a combination of free T3 levels in conjunction with symptoms of hypothyroidism, rather than looking just at the TSH. A key tenet of functional medicine is to get hormones into their optimal range, rather than just within the "normal" range. A suboptimal (bottom half of the normal range) T3 level with the patient's symptoms (including poor wound healing) is very suggestive of thyroid problems.

There is a variety of problems including obesity, inflammation, chronic illness, infection, and problems with adrenal function that inhibit the proper conversion of T4 to T3 in the periphery, although not necessarily in the brain. If you have a chronic wound, you almost surely have one or more of these issues.

Many physicians treat thyroid deficiency with only synthetic versions of thyroxine called Synthroid™ (levothyroxine.) Many patients on levothyroxine may normalize their TSH levels and be told they are "fine" despite having persistent symptoms of hypothyroidism. A much better solution in these patients is to treat them with natural desiccated thyroid (NDT). Most NDT preparations are of porcine (pig) origin and have both T3 and T4. It can change lives.

Many doctors are not familiar with a hormone called reverse T3 (rT3). It is made from T4 and blocks thyroid hormone receptors but does not activate them. This mechanism to turn down thyroid stimulation occurs for a variety of reasons, including adrenal dysfunction, diabetes, and iron deficiency. An elevated rT3 with respect to T3 levels (the T3/rT3 ratio is commonly used) can contribute to functional hypothyroidism. Many physicians have never even heard of rT3 and are not familiar with managing the level.

Hypothyroidism diagnoses are rising throughout the developed world; one reason is an increase in a condition called Hashimoto's thyroiditis. This autoimmune condition is associated with antibodies to thyroid peroxidase (TPO), an important enzyme in the thyroid gland. The most common causes of Hashimoto's are related to gluten sensitivity or other problems within the gut; thus, it can be improved by fixing one's diet and/or gut issues. It takes the right doctor to direct patients down this pathway.

Like all hormones, thyroid hormone has an appropriate optimal range— "more is not better." Being above the optimal range can cause as significant a problem as being significantly below it. Your thyroid hormone levels must be appropriately monitored and treated.

If you have a non-healing wound and you are not on thyroid replacement, or if you are on Synthroid or levothyroxine, have your TSH, free T3, free T4, and reverse T3 checked. If your free T3 is not in the top quartile, you may warrant treatment with a natural desiccated thyroid preparation. This should be considered in conjunction with your diurnal cortisol levels, TSH, free T4, and rT3. You may need to specifically seek out a knowledgeable physician for this. Finally, direct application of compounded T3 to wounds also stimulates wound healing.

CORTISOL

Cortisol is one of the few hormones that generally increases with age, and that is *not* a good thing. The pituitary gland (in the brain) produces adrenocortico-tropic hormone (ACTH), which stimulates the adrenal glands to produce cortisol. The actions of cortisol include raising blood sugar (to increase and store available energy [often as fat]), suppressing the immune system, stim-

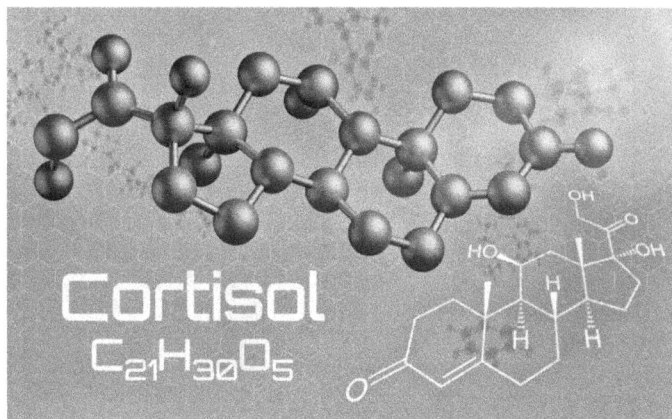

Cortisol
$C_{21}H_{30}O_5$

ulating alertness, and increasing sensitivity to adrenaline (epinephrine) and norepinephrine—essentially priming the body for the "fight or flight" response. Chronically disordered cortisol not only has a significant effect on the production of thyroid hormone but also directly affects wound healing.

Cortisol has a normal diurnal circadian rhythm—it rises early in the morning to wake you up. It usually peaks around 9:00 or 10:00 a.m. Production is shut down by morning sunlight, and it drops throughout the rest of the day until it is at its lowest right before bedtime. If your cortisol axis is functioning correctly, you should feel awake and energetic in the mornings and wind down and be able to get to sleep at night.

The best way to measure your cortisol is by getting levels at four or five different times during the day; this allows evaluation of your circadian rhythms. These tests are usually done on either saliva or dried urine and can be done in the privacy of your own home. It is important that you find a doctor who is knowledgeable about ordering and interpreting these tests.

Hypothalamic - Pituitary - Adrenal Axis

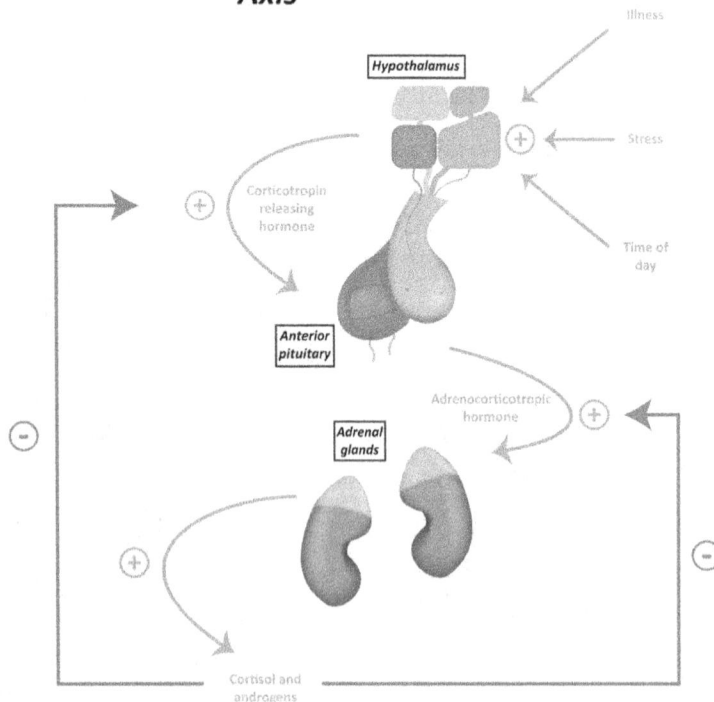

Anybody who is under chronic stress (and what is more stressful than having a chronic wound?) may be suffering from hypothalamic pituitary adrenal (HPA) axis dysfunction, previously known as "adrenal fatigue." When the brain is overwhelmed by having too much cortisol around for too long a time, it essentially shuts down cortisol production. When that occurs, the results include a lack of energy, foggy thinking, depression, chronic fatigue, poor wound healing, and a variety of other symptoms.

The treatments for both high and low cortisol include a special class of herbal medications known as adaptogens, which normalize the cortisol level whether it is high or low. These include rhodiola, ashwaganda, eleuthero, ginseng, licorice, astralgus, tulsi, and others. Those with high cortisol will also benefit from mindfulness techniques (meditation, yoga, prayer, Tai-Chi, Qigong, etc.). If your cortisol is low, you may also benefit from adrenal extracts and additional water-soluble B-vitamins and adequate trace minerals. In some cases, pharmaceutical grade hydrocortisone may be necessary.

Whether your cortisol is high or low (or normal) you need to pay strict attention to the circadian biology we have already discussed and make sure you are getting plenty of sleep and adequate amounts of sunlight, particularly in the mornings. Cortisol issues take at least six months and may take as long as two years to fix, but there is hope for getting them fixed and moving farther down the pathway to healing yourself and your wounds.

HUMAN GROWTH HORMONE

Human growth hormone (HGH), als important hormone secreted in pulsatile fashion by the pituitary gland after adequate melatonin production has been sensed. Although not all the effects are understood, we know HGH has many critical functions. Some of these include regulating metabolism, body composition (percent muscle

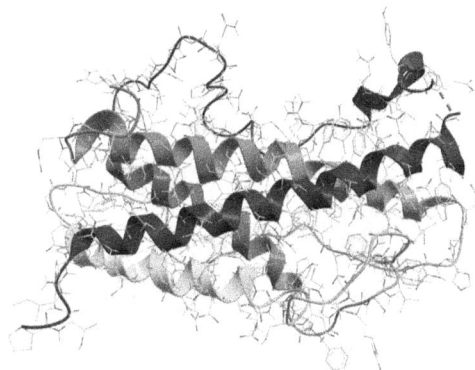

Molecular structure of
Human Growth Hormone

versus fat), glucose metabolism/production, promoting cell growth and division, promoting protein synthesis, and dealing with stress. It is critical to cellular repair processes including, not surprisingly, wound healing.

HGH has been shown to improve wound and bone healing when applied topically and when given systemically. Mechanisms by which it improves wound healing include stimulating granulation tissue formation, collagen deposition, and facilitating epithelialization (laying down of new skin). The increased anabolic (building/repairing) activity requires adequate amounts of protein intake.

Because HGH has been abused to enhance athletic performance, it has been very tightly regulated by the Food and Drug Administration in the United States. The only accepted use is to treat children with short stature. Although there is a recognized "adult onset growth hormone deficiency syndrome," the exact diagnosis requires not only symptom questionnaires but provocative testing that can be potentially dangerous to the patient. For these reasons, and the fact that it is quite expensive, HGH is rarely prescribed in the United States.

HGH release is triggered from the pituitary gland by growth hormone-releasing hormone (GHRH), which is secreted from the hypothalamus after adequate melatonin production has been sensed. There are some GHRH-like medications available, the most common of which is sermorelin. These medications are more available, less costly, and can be administered without the potential legal/compliance issues of HGH. Sermorelin has been anecdotally reported to improve wound healing, but there are few studies on it at this time. Although it is not strictly a "bioidentical" hormone, it has the same structure of the active part of the GHRH protein. We consider it a "last-line" agent for wound healing. Do everything else described in this book first, and you likely will not need it.

There are many things one can do to naturally increase HGH levels. Most importantly, optimize ocular melatonin synthesis during daylight hours (get the sun on your retinas—though, if you have had cataract surgery or have artificial lenses, this can be problematic), and make sure to protect your eyes and skin from light (especially blue light) after sundown to maximize melatonin secretion. Replacing/augmenting testosterone in both genders can also increase HGH secretion.

Other measures that help:

1. Lose excess body fat

2. Exercise

3. Fast intermittently

4. Reduce sugar intake

5. Do not eat within four hours of bedtime

6. Do high-intensity interval training (we realize this may not be something you can do easily … yet)

7. Consider supplementation with gamma-aminobutyric acid (GABA), arginine, and/or beta-alanine

But, by far, the most important way to maximize HGH production is to optimize your sleep time.

PREGNENOLONE

The next few hormones we discuss are called "steroid hormones," as their chemical structure is based on what is called a steroid molecule, a specific backbone of seventeen carbon atoms arranged in three six-atom rings and one five-atom ring. The most common steroid in the body is cholesterol, and from cholesterol is synthesized both active vitamin D (cholecalciferol) and pregnenolone.

Pregnenolone is known as the "mother hormone" because the remainder of the steroid hormones are synthesized from it. These include cortisol, aldosterone (important for salt and water balance in the body), DHEA, and the "sex steroid" hormones, which are testosterone, progesterone, and estrogen.

A common problem in those with chronic illness and wounds is "pregnenolone steal" syndrome. Pregnenolone is the substrate from which either cortisol or the important sex steroid hormones is made. Because of its evolutionary importance to survival, the production of cortisol is prioritized over the sex steroid hormones. In conditions of chronic stress (like a nonhealing wound), much of the available pregnenolone may be shunted down the cortisol pathway, and not enough is available to synthesize the other important hormones.

Like most of these hormones, pregnenolone levels can be tested, and, in the United States, pregnenolone is available over the counter, although as usual, buyer beware. It is possible to overuse it, and many OTC preparations do not contain exactly what they say they do.

If you have a chronic wound or non-healing wound, you should have your pregnenolone levels tested and consider supplementation to the top quartile. Although the specific effects of pregnenolone on wound healing have been only sparsely studied, it stands to reason that having enough pregnenolone around will improve wound healing, and indeed, we have found this to be the case. If you are on statin drugs to decrease your cholesterol—not something we are fans of—you may also find that you have very low pregnenolone levels.

DEHYDROEPIANDROSTERONE (DHEA)

DHEA is a steroid hormone made primarily by the adrenal glands. Although not all its functions are known or understood, production declines after age thirty and declines faster in some than others. It is a precursor to androgens and estrogens. Low DHEA levels correlate with higher risks for heart disease, cognitive decline, osteopenia, depression, and a host of other conditions. Assuring adequate DHEA levels is one of the mainstays of anti-aging medicine. DHEA levels can be measured in the blood, urine, or saliva, and most benefit from having it in the top quartile of the range of DHEA.

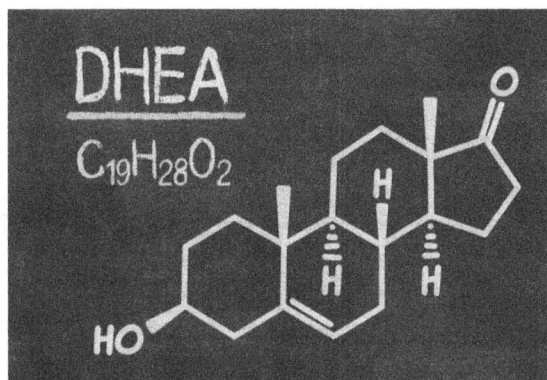

DHEA acts in wound healing by downstream activation of estrogenic receptors. A 2005 paper in the *Journal of Investigative Dermatology* showed that increased systemic levels of DHEA were protective against venous ulcers. In addition, local injection of DHEA accelerates impaired wound healing.

Have your DHEA level tested and supplement as needed to maintain upper quartile levels. Although side effects at levels modestly over the optimal range are uncommon, it is still better to test and dose accordingly. In the United States, DHEA is available over the counter, but as always, we favor pharmaceutical grade products for reliability.

How Hormones Are Made in Your Body

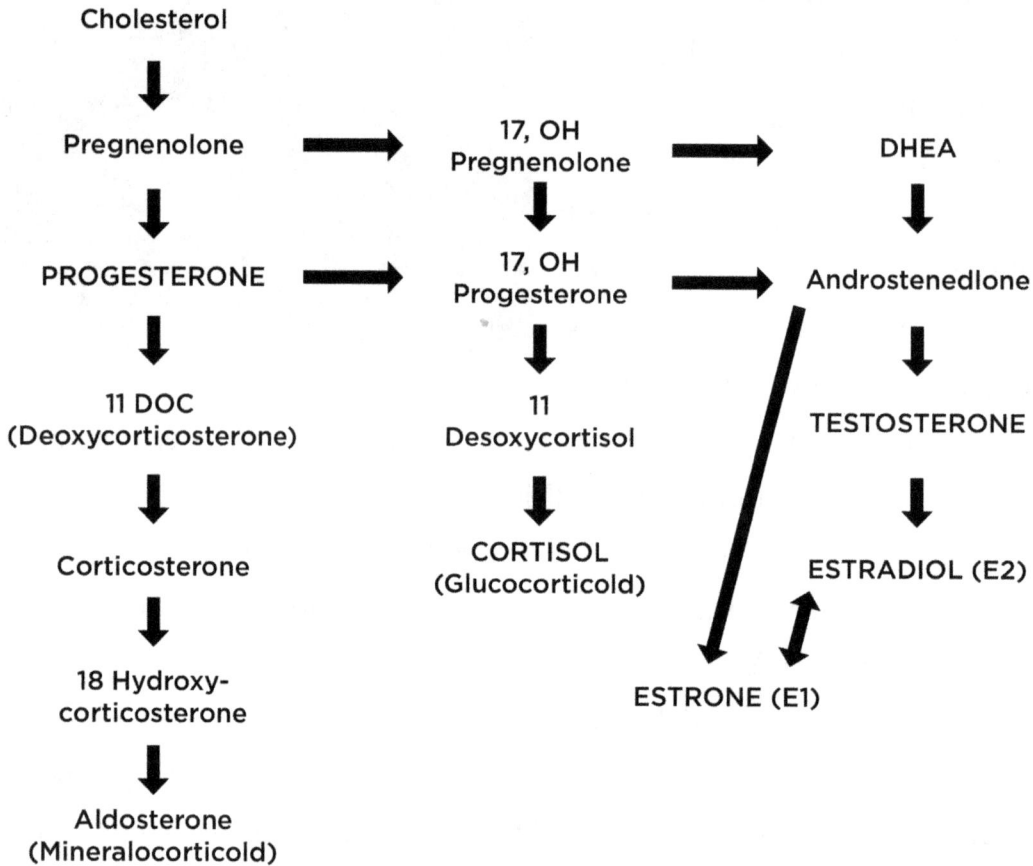

Cholesterol
↓
Pregnenolone → 17, OH Pregnenolone → DHEA
↓ ↓ ↓
PROGESTERONE → 17, OH Progesterone → Androstenedione
↓ ↓ ↓
11 DOC (Deoxycorticosterone) | 11 Desoxycortisol | TESTOSTERONE
↓ ↓ ↓
Corticosterone | CORTISOL (Glucocorticoid) | ESTRADIOL (E2)
↓ ↕
18 Hydroxy-corticosterone | ESTRONE (E1)
↓
Aldosterone (Mineralocorticoid)

TESTOSTERONE

Testosterone is found in both men and women. Although primarily thought of as the "male" hormone, during reproductive years it is actually present in women in a higher concentration than estradiol, which is the primary "female" hormone. In men, testosterone is primarily made by the testes, and in women, testosterone is made by both the ovaries and the adrenal glands.

Testosterone is an anabolic hormone—"anabolic" substances promote growth (and thus healing) and "catabolic" substances promote breakdown. You have probably heard of anabolic steroids; they are synthetic versions of testosterone that are modified to produce stronger or varied binding to hormone receptors to create specific effects like increased muscle mass. We do not prescribe nor recommend anabolic steroids, but we do prescribe bioidentical (the same as the human body makes) testosterone for both men and women.

As men age, testosterone levels naturally decrease. The rate of that decrease has substantially accelerated over the last fifty years or so. Many men in their forties (and even thirties) now have testosterone levels as low as they were in eighty-year-old men years ago. While the exact reasons for this are not well understood, we believe it is a combination of disordered circadian cycling, inflammation, environmental toxins, poor diets, inadequate nutrition, non-native EMF, and likely a variety of other factors. There is a plethora of likely contributing causes.

Testosterone Production Rate Declines by Age

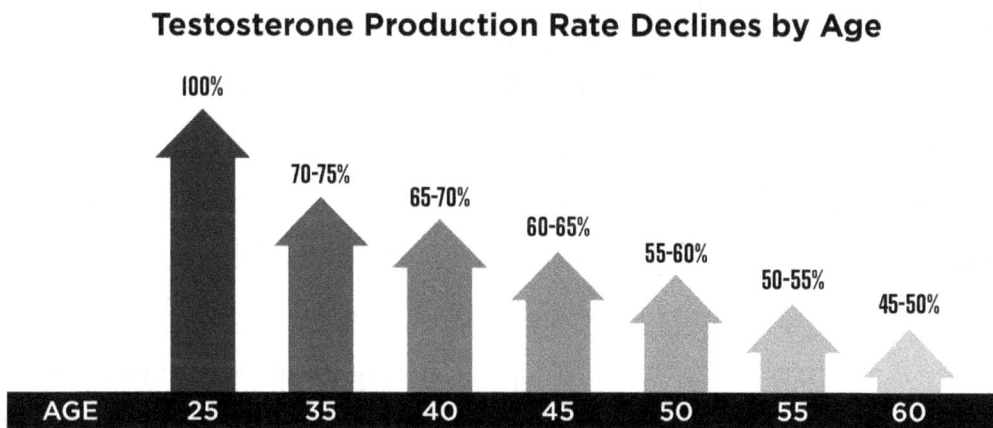

AGE	25	35	40	45	50	55	60
	100%	70-75%	65-70%	60-65%	55-60%	50-55%	45-50%

As testosterone declines in a man, more than just his libido suffers. So called "andropause" is associated with a variety of signs and symptoms including worsening body composition (more fat, less muscle), moodiness, irritability, poor sleep, skin aging and thinning, hair loss, osteoporosis, decreased muscular strength—including the all-important cardiac muscle—poor thinking, decreased ambition and goal-setting ability, worsening lipid panel, increased inflammation, poor blood sugar control, depression, anxiety, lethargy, etc. You get the picture. Receptors for this critically important hormone are found on every cell in the male body, and a deficiency of it has a tremendous effect on male health, including, not surprisingly, wound healing.

Diabetics are at particular risk for low testosterone and benefit greatly from testosterone replacement. It makes a tremendous difference to their overall health and well-being in addition to their wound healing capacity. Both systemic and topical testosterone (and even testosterone injected into the area of the wound) can have a tremendous effect on wound healing.

As women enter menopause, sex steroid hormone production decreases, starting with testosterone and followed sequentially by progesterone and estrogen. As a woman's natural testosterone levels decrease, a variety of symptoms sometimes just attributed to "aging" can often be alleviated by hormone replacement. These range from poor sleep, poor skin tone, moodiness, irritability, depression, anxiety, osteoporosis, decreased muscle tone, increased body fat, poor lipid panels, decreased libido, etc. Many of the symptoms are similar to what men experience and, of course, poor wound healing.

Replacing initially testosterone, then sequentially progesterone, then estrogen, often makes a huge difference in overall health, well-being, and wound healing for peri- or postmenopausal women.

There is a variety of methods to replace or augment testosterone levels in both men and women, each with its own advantages and disadvantages. We recommend you seek out a qualified anti-aging doctor to help you with this.

ESTROGEN AND PROGESTERONE

You may be familiar with "hot flashes" as the most common symptom of menopause, but there are many others, including mood swings, irritability, poor thinking, vaginal dryness, disturbed sleep, loss of muscle tone, depression, anxiety, and more. For years, women were placed on synthetic preparations of both estrogen (example: Premarin™) and progesterone (example: Provera™) to help alleviate these symptoms.

Studies have shown many benefits of postmenopausal hormone replacement in women, including decreased risk of cardiovascular disease, osteoporosis, dementia, an improved sense of well-being, sleep, libido, and mood. However, the synthetic hormones often carry undesirable side effects and have been shown to substantially increase the risk of cancer. For that reason, we only prescribe bioidentical hormones, which, when managed correctly, confer all the benefits but none of the risks.

In women, as progesterone and estrogen levels naturally decline, the ability to heal both acute and chronic wounds decreases. The exact mechanisms by which these hormones promote wound repair is still under study but appears to involve activation of various cells in the immune system and collagen deposition. Estrogen receptors have been found in nearly every cell in the female body, and estrogen is known to have over four hundred functions alone in the female body. Both progesterone and estrogen, both topically and systemically, have been shown to promote wound healing in post- and perimenopausal women.

HORMONE REPLACEMENT

Delving into the specifics of optimal hormone levels, delivery methods, and the advantages and disadvantages thereof is beyond the scope of this work; there are dozens of volumes available on this topic alone. The Internet abounds with information of varying quality about hormone replacement therapy. This is a complex field, and there are some potential risks to doing things wrong but also tremendous benefits to doing things right.

There are optimal ranges for most hormones (usually the top quartile, or one-fourth of the "normal range" that a lab reports out) and getting levels significantly above those can result in unwanted side effects or even cause medical problems. Hormone replacement should be undertaken carefully, with frequent monitoring, repeated laboratory testing for levels, and careful management of symptoms and dosage.

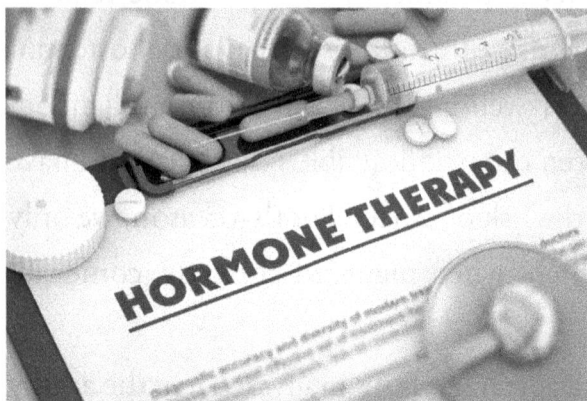

There is a variety of ways to replace or augment sex steroid hormone levels, including topical, oral, sublingual, injectable, or pellets. Each has benefits and potential problems, so we absolutely recommend you seek out a qualified practitioner to partner with you. With the right physician, you will be able to optimize and balance hormone levels and experience the many other benefits of bioidentical hormone replacement in addition to optimizing your wound healing.

If you make many (or all) of the lifestyle modifications we have discussed in this book, your hormone levels will improve significantly. However, if you have a non-healing wound, it is likely that you will need some significant help and external intervention (i.e. hormone replacement) to really initiate the healing process. Sometimes as you attain a state of better health, you will be able to decrease your hormone dosages and eventually wean off of them, although it is likely that as you age, your best chance of maintaining optimal health will involve careful bioidentical hormone replacement since we all lose these vital substances with the passage of time.

The bottom line is this: If you are over thirty and you have a chronic wound, find a qualified physician to help you get your hormones tested. Consider carefully the generally significant benefits versus the small risks of replacing your sex steroid hormones (testosterone, estrogen, and progesterone) and others if indicated by suboptimal levels.

References and Recommended Reading

1. Holick, M.F. *The Vitamin D Solution*. Carlton North, Vic.: Scribe, 2010. Print.

2. Bowthorpe, Janie A. *Stop the Thyroid Madness: A Patient Revolution against Decades of Inferior Thyroid Treatment*. Fredericksburg, TX: Laughing Grape Pub., 2012. Print.

3. Bowthorpe, Janie A., et al. *Stop the Thyroid Madness II: How Experts Are Challenging Ineffective Treatments and Improving the Lives of Patients*. Dolores, CO: Laughing Grape Pub. 2014. Print.

4. Wilson, Jim. *Adrenal Fatigue: The 21st Century Stress Syndrome*. Lanham: Smart Publications, 2010. Print.

5. Crisler, John. *Testosterone Replacement Therapy: A Recipe for Success*. United States: Milestones, 2014. Print.

6. Morgentaler, Abraham. *Testosterone for Life*. New York: McGraw-Hill, 2009. Print.

7. Maupin, Kathy C. *Secret Female Hormone: How Testosterone Replacement Can Change Your Life*. Carlsbad, CA: Hay House, 2015. Print.

8. Demling, R.H. "The Role of Anabolic Hormones for Wound Healing in Catabolic States." *Journal of Burns and Wounds*. 2005; 4: e2.

CHAPTER 10

Supplement Yourself

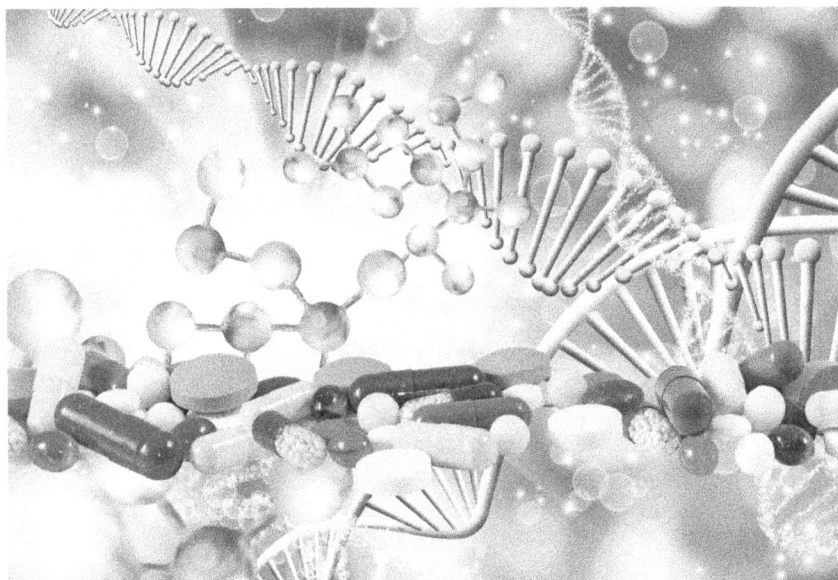

If we lived ideal lifestyles in a perfect world, none of us would need supplements, and in fact our goal is to get you to the place where you do not need them. However, if you have a non-healing wound, we are certain you need some extra help, and that is where dietary supplementation can be important.

As opposed to pharmaceuticals (medications), which are often patented, specialized synthetic compounds (although some are derived from natural sources), supplements are generally purified natural substances that can usually be bought over-the-counter (OTC). There are various types of supplements including necessary co-factors like vitamins and minerals, metabolic substrates for biochemical reactions, medicinal substances derived from plants, and hormones (such as vitamin D, DHEA, and adrenal extracts, previously discussed). While there are dozens (hundreds?) that have been described and found to have value, we will focus on the ones we have found to be the most helpful for our patients with non-healing wounds.

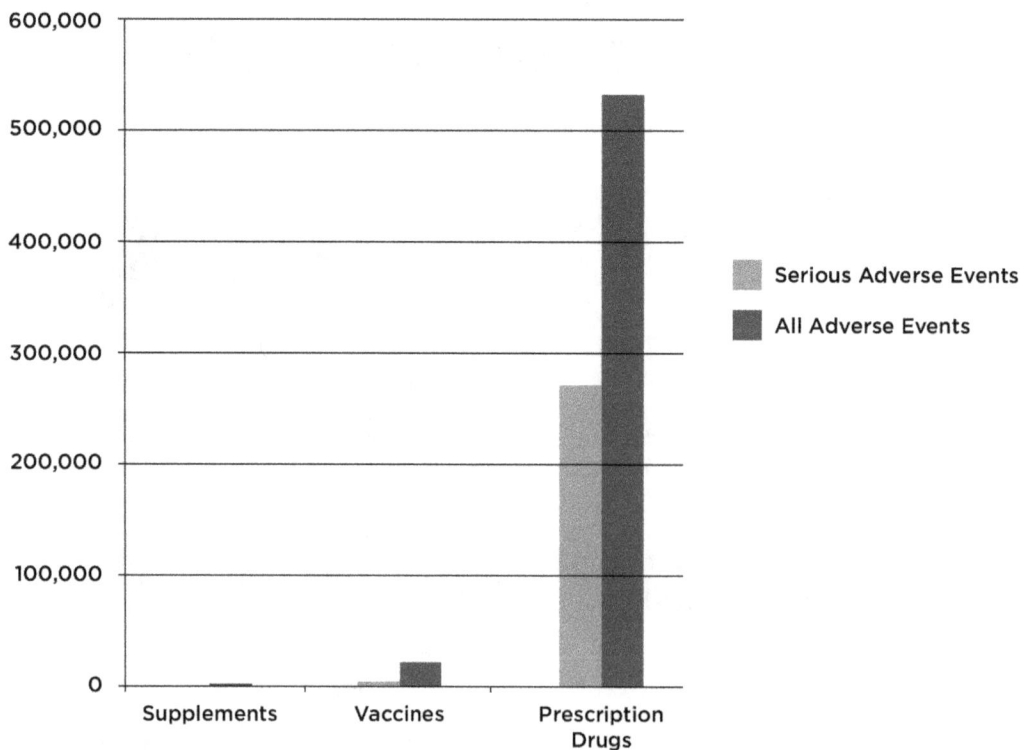

Purchase only top-quality, pharmaceutical grade supplements directly from reputable suppliers or manufacturers (we trust Pharmanex, Orthomolecular, Metagenics, Pure Encapsulations, and Douglas Labs, among others). In addition, we have created our own special line of supplements designed specifically to help with wound healing. Many supplements purchased in retail stores are counterfeit or have been improperly stored (this can be particularly true with bargain online sources). This may contribute to a lack of potency and efficacy, so if you are not sure what you are getting or cannot get the best ones, don't bother.

Almost all supplements should be taken with food. We are designed to absorb many of these substances from what we eat, and so it is important that they are absorbed along with many of the other beneficial substances that come in our (hopefully very high quality) diet. Your body was not designed/ evolved to take just a single substance at a time in a capsule. Notable exceptions are certain medications and hormones.

DHA—DOCOSAHEXAENOIC ACID—AN OMEGA-3 FATTY ACID

We discussed DHA previously in the nutrition chapter. The usual source is fish oil. By far, the best source of DHA is wild caught seafood, followed by grass fed meats and wild game. If you are a vegetarian or vegan (a bad idea—get checked for iron-deficiency anemia, B12 deficiency, and have an omega-3/ omega-6 fatty acid ratio test, among others …), alpha-linolenic acid (found in flax and chia seeds) can be somewhat helpful as a small percentage of it can be converted to DHA in your body—not enough though.

Many studies have correlated high tissue DHA levels with general health, along with decreased cardiovascular and neurodegenerative disease. However, like vitamin D and sunshine, supplementing with fish oil alone has not shown the same results. The literature on fish oil is somewhat contradictory regarding wound healing; it has potent anti-inflammatory properties and can slow the healing of acute wounds; however, all chronic wounds are stuck in an inflammatory phase and it can help move them through it. If you have a non-healing wound (and accompanying chronic illness), we suggest you supplement with quality, mercury-free fish oil. Take at least two grams a day, with meals. Refrigerate or freeze it to decrease problematic oxidation. Most importantly, eat more seafood.

VITAMINS AND MINERALS

Although many studies have questioned the value of multivitamins, our unqualified answer for those with non-healing wounds is yes. A *pharmaceutical grade* and complete multivitamin provides many of the cofactors necessary for critical chemical reactions in your body.

An optimal multivitamin is *not* going to be a single tablet, capsule, soft chew, or "gummy chew." You will need a combination of several capsules with doses well above the U.S. Recommended Daily Amount (RDA—the minimum to keep you alive and without deficiency diseases—not enough to restore your health).

Some of the most important micronutrients implicated in wound healing and worth additional supplementation:

- **Zinc** is required by over three hundred different enzymes for a variety of functions including DNA synthesis, cell division, protein synthesis, and collagen formation. Most good quality multivitamins will include an adequate amount of zinc. High dose oral zinc sulfate, 220 mg, three times a day, may speed healing time for some wounds by up to 43 percent.

- **Vitamin C (ascorbic acid)** deficiency famously causes scurvy, a deficiency disease in which connective tissue is weakened because of vitamin C's importance in collagen formation. Collagen is essential scaffolding for most tissues and thus necessary for wound healing. Humans lack the ability to store vitamin C, so having an adequate dietary amount is important. It is also an important antioxidant that counteracts the potentially harmful reactive oxygen species found in wounds. Suggested dose of vitamin C is 2,000 mg per day until your wound is healed, then 1,000 mg per day thereafter.

- **Vitamin A** enhances the early inflammatory phase of wound healing. It is required for epithelial (skin) tissue differentiation and immune system function. It improves collagen cross-linking and wound breaking strength. Because vitamin A is fat soluble it is (rarely) possible to build up to toxic levels with prolonged mega-dosing. Safe dosing is 25,000 IU per day for three months to facilitate wound healing.

However, one very important mineral that you must watch out for is iron. If your body's iron stores are too high it can lead to very serious problems. It is very important to have your doctor check your ferritin level and if higher than the optimal range of 40-70 ng/ml then you should be either donating blood periodically or having therapeutic phlebotomy. See the book on iron cited in our resource section for further details.

METHYLATION

Approximately 40 percent of the general population, including most of our wound patients, has a mutation in genes coding for enzymes for "methylation." Methylation is critical to a variety of processes including activating and deactivating hormones, neurotransmitters, and gene transcription. It is also necessary for detoxifying some substances.

Those with methylation defects benefit from methylated B vitamins including methyl-cobalamin (B12), methyltetrahydrofolate (B6), and tri-methyl glycine (TMG, also known as betaine). These are usually sold in combination "methylation supplements." Ask your doctor about being tested for methylation defects. If you have not been (or cannot be) tested and are not sure if you have a methylation defect, you should take a methylation supplement at least until your wound heals. When possible, get tested and if you do have a methylation problem, then you should plan on taking a methylation supplement for life. This makes a huge difference in your current and future health and decreases your risk for numerous problems including migraines, allergies, asthma, cardiovascular disease, cancer, and others.

THE MITOCHONDRIAL PRESCRIPTION

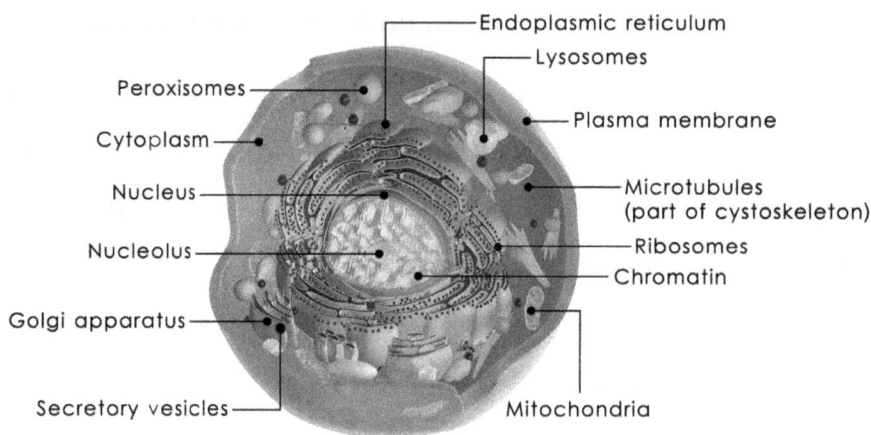

Mitochondria are tiny organelles in your cells that are essentially power plants. Without the right mitochondrial substrates, you cannot heal. One of the primary functions of mitochondria is to produce adenosine triphosphate (ATP), known as the energy currency of the cell. A cell with abundant ATP and energy is healthy and vital, but a cell without energy is … dead! Effective mitochondrial function is at the root of *all* health.

The following supplements, taken together, constitute a "mitochondrial prescription" and are important for at least a six-month period if you have a chronic wound.

- **Magnesium** has three different magnesium formulations. Magnesium threonate (2,000 mg twice per day) is most helpful to the brain and spinal cord. Magnesium maleate (1,250 mg twice per day) is preferred by skeletal muscles, and magnesium orotate (300-500 mg twice per day) is best for cardiac muscle. Magnesium is critical for optimal mitochondrial function. Magnesium deficiency is widespread, especially in diabetics. It also plays an important role in sugar metabolism. High magnesium diets and supplementation significantly decrease the risks of developing type 2 diabetes. Magnesium supplementation is safe unless you have end stage renal disease and are on dialysis. If so, discuss with your physician.

- **Taurine** is naturally found in seafood and meat, and it helps maintain the pH gradient across the mitochondrial membrane. Take 2,000 mg per day. Vegans/vegetarians are particularly likely to have taurine deficiency.

- **D-ribose** is a five-carbon sugar that serves as a (recyclable) building block of ATP. D-ribose is important for cellular energy production and is particularly helpful in heart failure. Take fifteen grams (yes, grams not milligrams) of D-ribose per day. Don't worry about the "sugar" content; it is not metabolized the same as dietary sugars like glucose and fructose and will not affect your blood sugar (glucose) levels.

- **Co-Q10** (coenzyme-Q10) is necessary for mitochondrial energy production and a critical part of electron chain transport. Of the available formulations, the "ubiquinol" form is preferred over "ubiquinone." Take 300 mg per day.

- **Acetyl L-carnitine** transfers carbon fragments from long-chain fatty acids across the inner mitochondrial membrane. L-carnitine improves lipid profiles by lowering LDL and raising HDL cholesterol, and the acetyl variety gets into the central nervous system. It is found in meats and seafood. Vegans, vegetarians, and those with kidney disease, B-vitamin deficiencies, and iron deficiency anemia are usually very deficient in L-carnitine. Acetyl L-carnitine promotes fatty acid metabolism in the hypoxic cellular environment typical of chronic wounds. Take 1,000 mg three times a day.

AMINO ACIDS

Proteins are made of chains of amino acids. Although we have discussed the importance of adequate protein intake (from whole food) for wound healing, sometimes specific amino acid supplementation for wounds can be very helpful.

- **Glutamine**. L-glutamine has been shown to be beneficial for both surgical and chronic wound healing. Ten grams a day is the suggested dose if you suffer from a chronic wound. It is prescribed to help heal "leaky gut" syndrome; it is quite effective at healing the intestinal lining.

- **Arginine**. L-arginine is important for nitric oxide synthesis in the body. Nitric oxide is an important vasodilator and stimulator of angiogenesis. It lowers blood pressure, improves tissue oxygenation, and helps heal wounds. The dose is five grams twice per day. If you have a history of herpes or shingles, it should be taken combined with two grams per day of L-lysine (another amino acid), which decreases the risk of an outbreak.

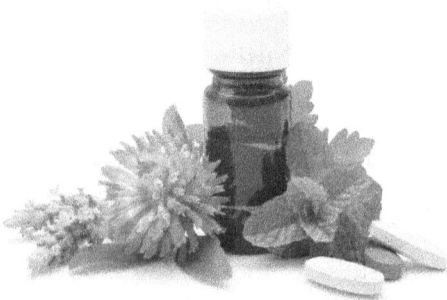

OTHER VALUABLE SUPPLEMENTS

Scientific studies are beginning to validate the efficacy and explore mechanisms of action for these botanical medicines.

- **Curcumin** is the active ingredient of turmeric, the main spice in curry dishes. There are over six thousand publications detailing beneficial effects. It is anti-inflammatory, anti-coagulant, anti-depressant, anti-cancer, and analgesic. It reverses insulin resistance, lowers blood sugar, and improves lipids. If you are going to take just one medicinal herb, this is it. We suggest using copious quantities in cooking and making turmeric tea. A small amount of black pepper increases the bioavailability. Suggested dose as a supplement is 2,000 mg per day.

- **Boswellia** is a potent anti-inflammatory used in traditional Ayurvedic medicine and promotes angiogenesis, the formation of new blood vessels, which is critical to wound healing. Supplement dose of 300 mg of the standardized extract two to three times per day.

- **Devil's claw** is an anti-inflammatory derived from a South African fruit, which has been shown to reduce the pain and inflammation of arthritis and has potent wound healing effects, both applied topically and taken internally. Supplement dose of 200–2,500 mg per day.

- **Berberine** is an alkaloid derived from a variety of plant sources (including goldenseal, Oregon grape, and barberry) that has been used in traditional medicine for hundreds of years. It improves immune function, glucose metabolism, insulin sensitivity, lipid metabolism, gastrointestinal function, and overall health. It is very beneficial to the cardiovascular system and has been shown to be as effective as the pharmaceutical metformin at decreasing blood sugar in diabetics. Additionally, it has been shown to have beneficial effects on wound healing. Take 500 mg two to three times per day.

- **Olive leaf extract** (oleopein) has been extensively studied and found to have anti-inflammatory, anti-infective and anti-neoplastic (anti-cancer) properties in addition to beneficial cardiovascular effects such as lowering blood pressure and improving arterial health. It is also a particularly effective natural broad-spectrum antibiotic that destroys both bacteria and viruses—great for helping infected wounds. Dose is 500 mg per day.

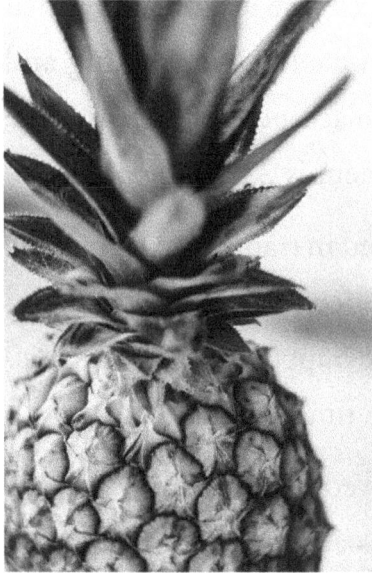

- **Bromelains** are a family of enzymes derived from the pineapple plant. Bromelain reduces edema, bruising, pain, and healing times following injuries and surgical procedures, and in chronic wounds. Bromelain has significant anti-inflammatory activity and increases the re-absorption of hematomas (collections of blood under the skin). Dose is 800–1,000 mg twice per day.

- **Alpha lipoic acid** is an important antioxidant that plays a significant role in glucose control. Taking 600 mg twice a day, an hour prior to eating, will be helpful for both wound healing and diabetes.

- **Chlorella** are algae from Japan and Taiwan which have numerous benefits including detoxifying heavy metals, improving immune function, decreasing blood sugar, and increasing cellular growth rates, which are a major factor in the natural repair of wounds. Chlorella helps heal ulcers and promotes bone and muscle growth. Buy "cracked cell wall" chlorella and take five to ten grams per day.

- **Gotu kola** (centella asiatica) has been used as a natural medicine for the treatment of scars and wounds across Asia for many centuries. Topical creams for your wounds are available. The oral dose is 250–500 mg three times per day.

- **Aloe vera** has been used for centuries, both topically and internally, to enhance wound repair (and a multitude of skin conditions).

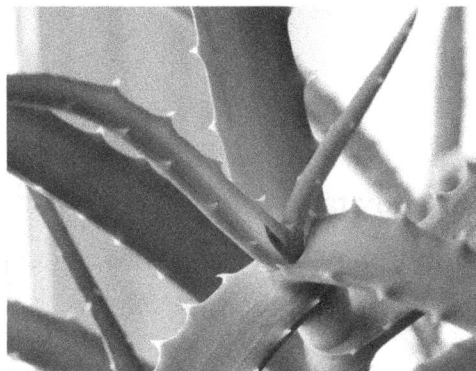

CONCLUSION

As you have seen, there are many supplements that have been shown to be helpful in wound healing. We have given you a list of more than a dozen possibilities here—so where should you start? You could potentially take all of them at once but that is a lot of capsules or pills to take daily, which is a huge nuisance, and frankly gets very expensive.

Here's how we recommend sequencing things:

- Make as many of the lifestyle changes as you can to optimize vitamin D and DHA. Have your vitamin D levels measured and supplement as needed. Commit to taking an excellent quality fish oil for at least a year or until your wound is healed. Of course, eat well as discussed in the chapter on nutrition.

- Take a good quality multivitamin as described earlier and a methylation supplement unless you are certain you do not have a methylation defect.

- Follow the "mitochondrial prescription" for at least six months.

- Choose two of the remaining compounds listed and take for at least three months. Rotate and choose another two and keep doing that.

- Look for combination products that contain more than one of the ingredients listed; for example, there is an excellent anti-inflammatory product available which contains turmeric, devil's claw, and Boswellia in appropriate doses.

The goal with appropriate lifestyle changes is to eventually get you off all but a few supplements (multivitamin and maybe a methylation supplement). However, in the short term it may be necessary to aggressively use supplements to heal your wound and regain your health.

Finally, there is a lot of fraud and poor products being sold in the supplement markets. If you are not getting some effects from your supplements, you either have some serious digestion and malabsorption issues or you are taking a poor-quality product. Make sure to buy pharmaceutical grade supplements from reputable suppliers, consider seeing an appropriate functional medicine physician for gut healing, and follow some of our prior guidelines to get your digestive tract working as optimally as possible.

References and Recommended Reading

1. MacKay DJ, and Alan LM. "Nutritional support for wound healing." *Alternative Medicine Review* Nov. 2003: 359+. *Academic OneFile.* Web. 24 Aug. 2016.

2. Mangan, P. D., and Leo Zacharski. *Dumping Iron: How to Ditch This Secret Killer and Reclaim Your Health.* North Charleston, SC: CreateSpace Independent Platform, 2016. Print.

3. Pories, W J et al. "Acceleration of Healing with Zinc Sulfate." *Annals of Surgery* 165.3 (1967): 432–436. Print.

4. Ringsdorf, W. M., George Manstein, and N. Cheraski. "Vitamin C and Human Wound Healing." *Plastic and Reconstructive Surgery* 70.5 (1982): 657. Web.

5. Hobson, Rachel. "Vitamin E and Wound Healing: An Evidence-based Review." *International Wound Journal* 13.3 (2014): 331–35. Web.

6. Mehraein, Fereshteh, Maryam Sarbishegi, and Anahita Aslani. "Evaluation of Effect of Oleuropein on Skin Wound Healing in Aged Male Balb/c Mice." *Cell Journal (Yakhteh)* 16.1 (2014): 25–30. Print.

7. Jalilimanesh M, Mozaffari-Khosravi H, and Azhdari M. "The Effect of Oral L-glutamine on the Healing of Second-degree Burns in Mice." *Wounds* 2011; 23 (3): 53–58.

8. Larsson SC, and Wolk A. "Magnesium intake and risk of type 2 diabetes: a meta-analysis." *J Intern Med.* 2007 Aug; 262(2): 208-14.

9. Yin J, Xing H, Ye J. "Efficacy of Berberine in patients with type 2 diabetes mellitus." *Metabolism.* May 2008; 57(5): 712–717.

10. Zhang Y, et al. "Treatment of type 2 diabetes and dyslipidemia with the natural plant alkaloid berberine." *J Clin Endocrinol Metab* . 2008; 93(7): 2559–65.

11. Chuengsamarn S, et al. "Curcumin extract for prevention of type 2 diabetes." *Diabetes Care.* 2012 Nov; 35(11): 2121–7.

CHAPTER 11

Unravel the Mystery
of Wound Healing

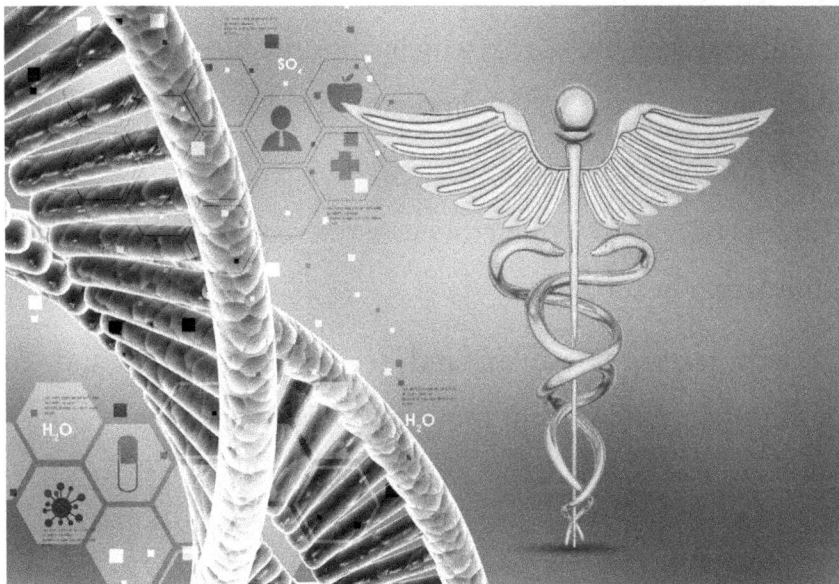

We all accept that kids heal much faster than adults, and hopefully by now you realize some of the reasons why. Is it any surprise that aging slows healing and that adults with chronic illnesses develop chronic wounds?

When you were a child and you fell off your bike and scraped your knee, your parents may have cleaned the wound and put a Band-Aid on it, but that is probably all they needed to do. Your body has built-in repair systems to take care of the damage. A scab develops and you form new skin beneath the scab.

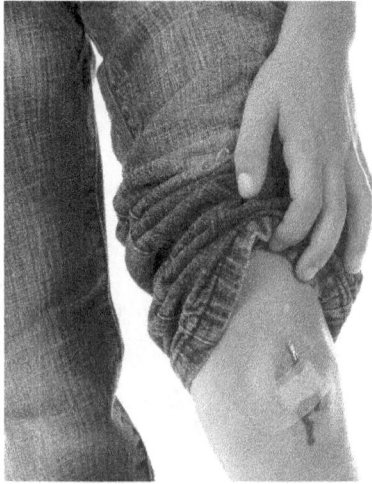

Although your age and various maladies, toxins, and stressors to your body have diminished that ability now, rest assured that you have not lost the ability to heal … not yet. Not when the wound is still acute.

Here is what happens right after an injury:

1. The injured tissue releases calcium, which signals to the platelets that damage has occurred.

2. Platelets respond by activating the thrombin cascade. The thrombin cascade causes a blood clot which stops the bleeding. This platelet rich fibrin matrix is the yellow goo you saw around your scab when you fell as a child.

3. Platelets release growth factors into the matrix, holding it in place and stimulating healing.

4. Growth factors stimulate and recruit both local and circulating multipotent stem cells to grow new, healthier tissue.

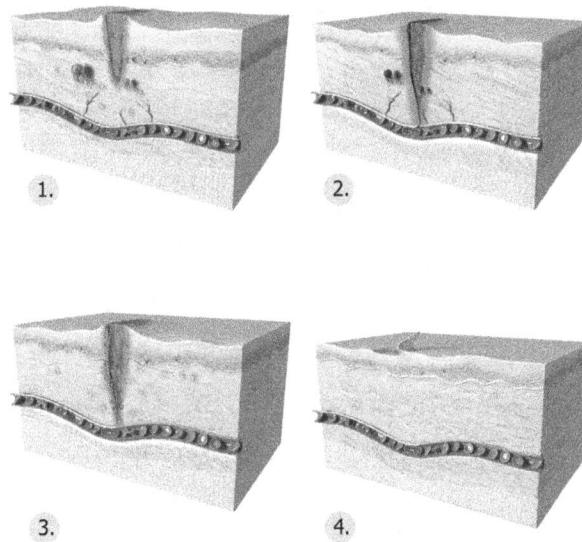

The four phases of normal wound healing

Here is a description of what differentiates normal from abnormal wound healing.

NORMAL WOUND HEALING

The healing process is initiated following a cut, scrape, or even a large surgical incision. This is a highly evolved process that we take for granted. Ordinarily, this occurs in a timely and sequential manner characterized by four distinct phases: coagulation, inflammation, proliferation, and remodeling. The complexity of interactions required to organize and achieve these steps will show that healing a wound is indeed miraculous.

Coagulation occurs immediately after injury to help minimize blood loss (a process called hemostasis). Blood vessels and capillaries (the smallest blood vessels) constrict (vasoconstriction) and platelets form clots to prevent blood loss and provide the matrix (scaffolding) for cell migration. Platelets also secrete growth factors. Chemicals called cytokines attract fibroblasts, endothelial cells, and immune cells. The matrix these cells provide is the initial phase of wound repair.

During the next phase, known as the inflammatory phase, dead cells, bacteria, and foreign matter (dust, grit, etc.) are removed by the white blood cells engulfing them and breaking them down through the bloodstream. This process by which a cell engulfs ("eats") something (bacteria, debris, etc.) is known as phagocytosis, and the primary phagocytic cells of the body are called neutrophils and macrophages. These help prevent bacterial contamination and cleanse the wound of cellular debris.

Platelets secrete various growth factors and cytokines, which recruit even more fibroblasts (cells that produce new skin and collagen), endothelial cells (which eventually turn into skin and the lining of blood vessels), and keratinocytes (which repair damaged blood vessels). During this time, cell division occurs to regrow tissue, leading to the proliferation phase. In a healthy wound (healthy person), the inflammatory phase should only last about seven days.

During the proliferative phase, local stem cells differentiate into necessary tissues to repair and rebuild the wound. They may help form new bone, tendon, muscle, subcutaneous tissue, or skin. This phase is characterized by granulation tissue (fibroblasts help form new tissue to fill in the defect), angiogenesis (formation of new blood vessels), and epithelialization (the formation of new skin). Wound closure marks the completion of this phase.

Remodeling is the final phase and can last a year or longer. During this phase, the skin matrix is remodeled into organized collagen bundles, and a scar forms. Some people form more prominent scars than others (keloids).

Young, healthy people with injuries typically follow these four phases of healing and have no need for a wound center. Most surgical incisions proceed through this orderly and timely sequence as well.

If your wound has not healed after three weeks (four weeks for very large wounds), it has transitioned to a "chronic wound," and the chance of it healing on its own decreases significantly. You will need to use some of the tips discussed in the following chapters. After three weeks if you still have a wound, and especially if there is drainage from the wound, the recommendations in this book are for you.

ABNORMAL WOUND HEALING

Chronic wounds have all failed to advance through these four normal phases of healing in the expected manner. They are usually stuck and remain stalled in the inflammatory phase. Examples include diabetic foot ulcers, venous leg ulcers, pressure ulcers, and some wounds from trauma or injury. Deterrents to normal healing include age, smoking, infection, ischemia (lack of adequate blood flow), edema, unrelieved pressure, or repetitive mechanical injury (pressure, rubbing, friction, abrasion, etc.). These wound environments are prohibitive to stem cells functioning correctly. Even if stem cells were initially recruited to the wound, they cannot differentiate and function normally. The clinical result is a non-healing wound due to excessive inflammation and (usually) persistent infection.

Chronic wounds have lost the ability to restore the soft tissue injury by regenerating tissue back to its former structure. They can only repair and replace it with the scarring process.

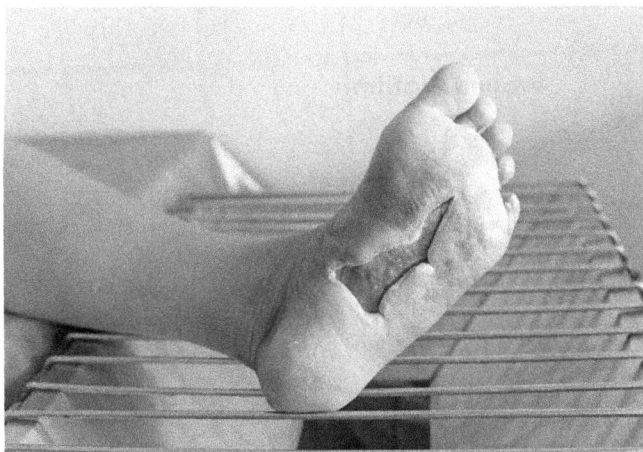

Chronic diabetic foot ulcer:
no similarities to the acute wound on page 132

While necessary for survival, this is not a good thing functionally. Scar tissue is less robust (this explains why ten to fifteen percent of all laparotomies result in a hernia). This also explains why so many wounds reoccur in the same location.

Chronic wounds develop drug-resistant biofilms, which you can think of as a nasty crust of bacteria, dead cells, and environmental contaminants (dust, lint, hair, dirt, etc.).

What is a biofilm? It is any group of microorganisms in which cells stick to each other and adhere to a surface. These cells become embedded within a matrix of extracellular polymeric substance; another (very descriptive) name for it is slime.

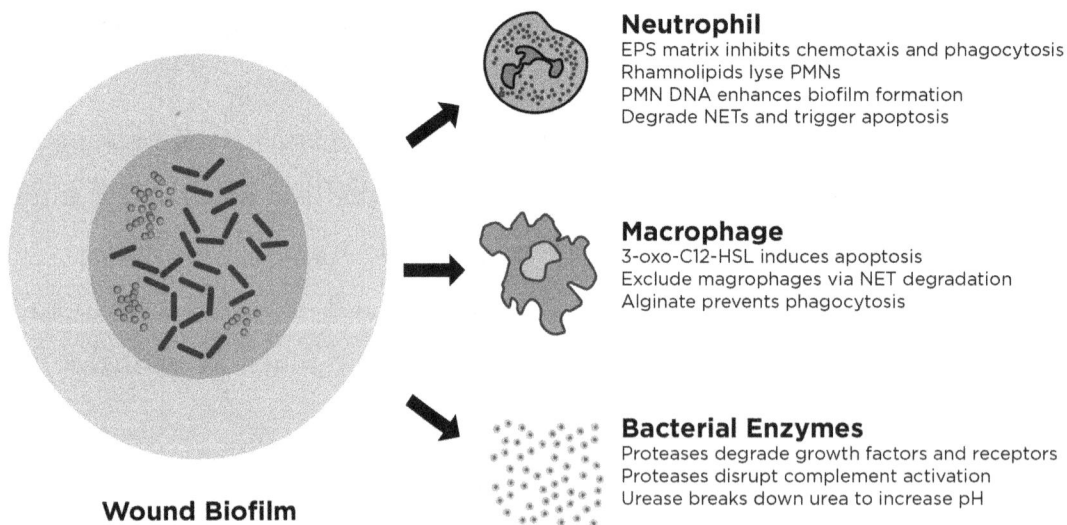

Neutrophil
EPS matrix inhibits chemotaxis and phagocytosis
Rhamnolipids lyse PMNs
PMN DNA enhances biofilm formation
Degrade NETs and trigger apoptosis

Macrophage
3-oxo-C12-HSL induces apoptosis
Exclude magrophages via NET degradation
Alginate prevents phagocytosis

Bacterial Enzymes
Proteases degrade growth factors and receptors
Proteases disrupt complement activation
Urease breaks down urea to increase pH

Wound Biofilm

Often, particularly on feet, another factor is constant or recurring pressure on the area (i.e. walking or standing). The tissue is hypoxic (has a relative lack of oxygen or a low oxygen level). Hypoxia increases the risk of local infection and retards tissue growth, catapulting the wound into a chronic and vicious cycle from which it is hard to emerge.

While the underlying pathology of diabetic foot ulcers, vascular ulcers, pressure ulcers, and non-healing surgical wounds may differ, hypoxia (inadequate amount of oxygen reaching the tissues) is at the core of them all. This is why hyperbaric oxygen therapy can be so effective and is used in many wound centers. HBOT increases the tissue levels of oxygen and helps a wound break out of this cycle (more in Chapter 17).

Almost every wound would benefit from HBOT (as an adjunct to conventional wound care). However, to control costs, insurers typically only approve HBOT for certain few wounds after other means have failed. In addition, there are frequently required waiting periods before HBOT can even be considered; this can be incredibly frustrating for both physicians and patients. Often HBOT would *reduce* overall costs since fewer visits to a wound center, fewer expensive biological dressings, and fewer surgeries (amputations) might result.

Keeping wounds moist leads to faster healing. Scabs (medical term: eschars) are barriers to healing a chronic wound. Eschar prevents the generation of new tissue and wound closure. Eschar layers (dead cells) can be carefully removed by a specialist to create a clean moist wound bed, allowing the tissue regenerative process to begin. This process is called debridement. Done correctly, healing time decreases, but just "picking" at the scabs can actually prolong healing time and increase the chance of scarring.

Many primary care providers prefer the "let it scab over" approach. They are often reluctant to refer the patient to a wound care center unless they suspect a severe infection or an abscess. We see the same with orthopedic surgeons and podiatrists. After repairing fractured bones or performing joint surgery, even if a patient develops a "fracture blister" or requires a wound vac because their surgical incision opened, they are not always referred to a wound center. Usually these patients are only referred after several visits (and one or more rounds of antibiotics) when it becomes clear that the wound is either not improving or worsening. Meanwhile under that firm, hypoxic eschar, or in that open, deshisced surgical wound, a deep space infection is brewing. If these patients were referred to a wound specialist early in their course, the patient could potentially have been spared weeks, if not months, of misery.

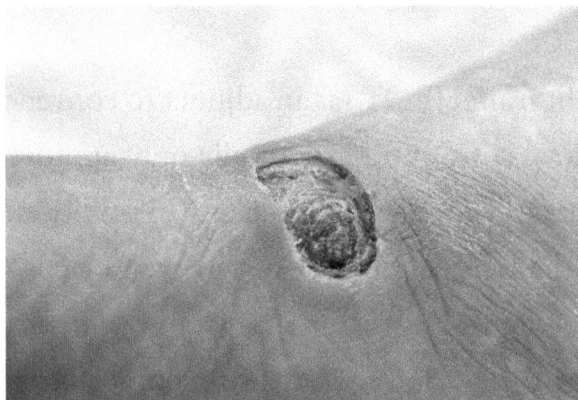

Wound from pressure injury which has now become a chronic ulcer

In our experience, changing the practice patterns of community doctors to make referrals to wound centers in a timely fashion has proven extremely challenging. Moreover, if you have a history of non-healing wounds, chances are that you are a poor healer and should not even wait a few weeks to return to the wound center.

PREVENTING WOUNDS

As with everything in medicine, prevention is key, and wounds are no exception. Dry skin is one of the biggest risks for developing wounds, especially pressure ulcers. When skin becomes dry, flaky, and fragile, it is more prone to ulcerating. Moisturizers may be needed (such as vitamin A and D, aquaphor, coconut oil, or urea). On the other hand, if skin is too moist (such as in skin folds, near and around the rectum, or around a draining wound), it becomes white and fragile (known as maceration). In those cases, barrier cream such as Calazime or vitamin A and D ointment with zinc is helpful to protect the skin.

If you (ever) develop swelling in your legs, this is critical to manage. Edema is one of the greatest risk factors predisposing you to skin infection, or cellulitis. It can cause microtears or blisters, which serve as entry ports for bacteria. When breaks in the skin occur and venous/lymphatic drainage is obstructed, bacteria are able to spread through the superficial tissues creating a localized area of infection. Areas of skin breakdown progress to ulceration.

Not only does the edema prevent the lymphatic system from clearing microbes that have breached the skin, but the impaired circulation limits the delivery of antibiotics to those tissues. If bacteria spread to the deeper tissues, an abscess (or worse) may develop.

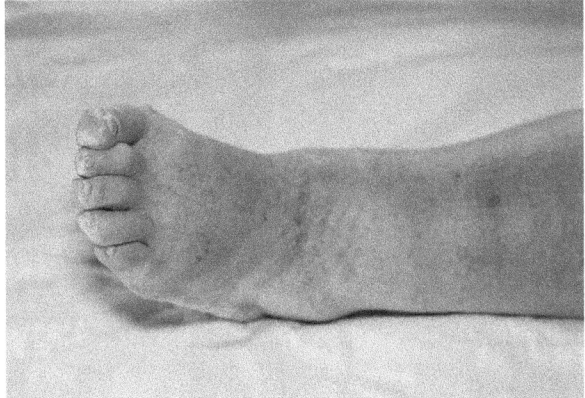

Risk factors for cellulitis include blockage in drainage return from venous insufficiency (or saphenous veinectomy in coronary artery bypass), breaks in the skin (trauma, ulceration, edema), inflammatory disease of the skin (allergic contact dermatitis, atopic dermatitis, venous eczema), older age, and diabetes. Obesity adds another risk factor due to the compression of the lymphatic flow by excess adipose tissue.

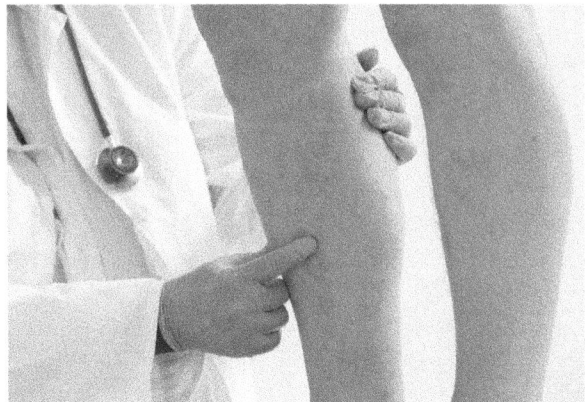

Varicose veins, an indicator of underlying chronic venous insufficiency, which predisposes skin to ulcerate unless treated

By far the best strategy to prevent chronic wounds is to avoid injury as much as possible, and if you do develop one to immediately identify and start appropriate treatment. It should go without saying that all the steps we have discussed previously with regard to optimizing your health are vital and far-reaching.

CHAPTER 12

Strategies to Help You Heal

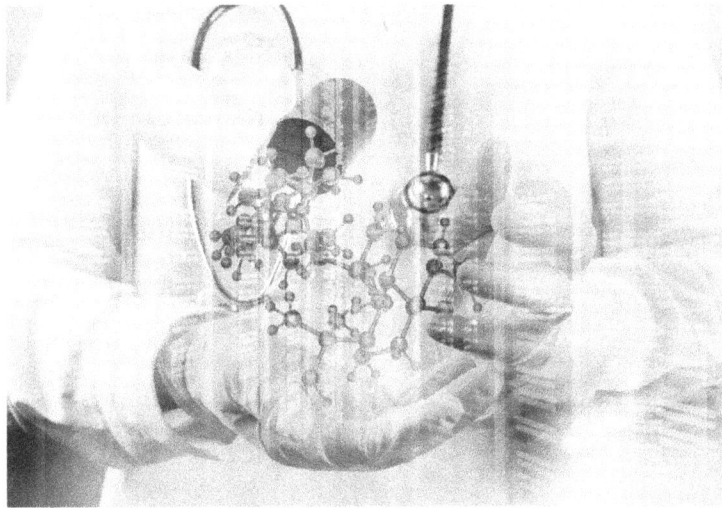

I. ACUTE WOUND CONSIDERATIONS

One of the most important considerations for acute wounds is whether or not you can take care of them yourself. The number of wound permutations and possibilities, along with potential associated injuries is nearly endless (we have seen most but certainly not all of them in the ER), so we will not presume to cover them all here. You should seek qualified care immediately for wounds with excessive bleeding; exposed tendons, bone, or subcutaneous tissue (fat); wounds over joints; or wounds that impair function (i.e. fingers/toes moving correctly). Wounds on the neck, chest, abdomen or pelvis are all potentially serious also.

Usually the most effective way to stop bleeding for acute wounds (and even chronic wounds that bleed when being cleaned) is direct pressure on the wound with a clean (better yet sterile) dressing material. Elevating the wound above the level of the heart can be helpful. If bleeding persists or you are on blood thinning medication (warfarin, Coumadin, Plavix, Xarelto, Eliquis, Pradaxa, or similar), then seek appropriate help. If your wound is bleeding badly enough that you need a tourniquet, you must seek help immediately!

Deep or full-thickness skin lacerations should be properly cleaned and, if necessary, closed (with staples or sutures) within six to eight hours. Delaying the time to closure significantly increases the risk of infection. After that, your doctor may not be willing to close your wound, and healing takes a lot longer.

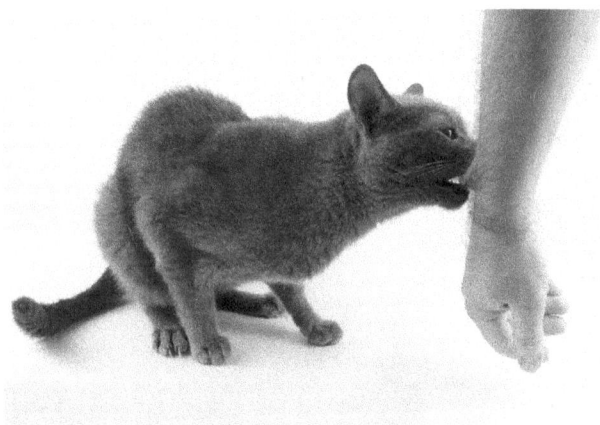

Bites (especially cat bites and human bites) are very concerning because of the multitude and virulence of the organisms present. Bites to the hands are at particularly high risk for infection of tendon and bone. Antibiotics are generally necessary. Likewise, deep puncture wounds, especially of the feet (and especially those made by something puncturing a shoe/sock) need to be cleaned immediately and thoroughly; they should be evaluated by a physician, and most circumstances require antibiotics. Sometimes x-rays or other imaging is necessary to find and remove foreign material.

142

Case Report: Puncture Wound

Mr. G, a type 2 diabetic, was repairing a fence on his ranch when he stepped on wire protruding from the ground. It penetrated his shoe and sock and became embedded in his heel. He did not have diabetic neuropathy and, fortunately, felt it right away. He removed his shoe and sock and then pulled the wire out. "It felt like it went into the bone." He went right to the local ER where x-rays did not show remaining wire or obvious bone problems. The wound was rinsed, and he was given a tetanus booster and prescribed antibiotics. He finished the antibiotics, but the pain with walking persisted, so he was prescribed a stronger course of antibiotics.

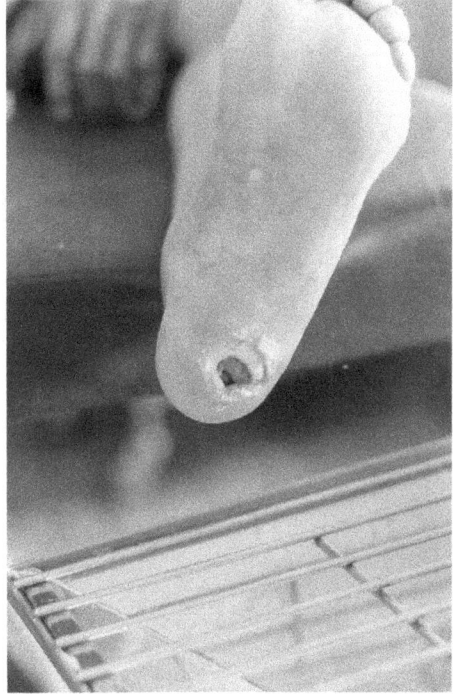

About three months later, he awakened with severe heel pain, was unable to bear weight, and noticed redness and swelling up to his ankle. X-rays confirmed chronic osteomyelitis, and a draining sinus tract from the infected bone had developed. After obtaining a bone culture, I ordered six weeks of intravenous antibiotics and HBOT and kept him off his foot with a knee-scooter. The infection resolved and the wound closed, and fortunately he made a complete recovery.

1. Cleaning Your Wound

The skin is your first line of defense against the environment. When it is not intact, a myriad of microbes (bacteria, fungi, viruses) can penetrate your body, causing infection that inhibits healing (or can even be life threatening). The most important thing you can do to prevent this is to properly clean wounds immediately after the injury. In the case of chronic wounds, unless instructed otherwise, daily cleansing is likewise important; it is like a minor debridement that helps remove the biofilm that inhibits healing.

To reduce the potential of worsening infection, wash your hands thoroughly before cleaning your wound. Use soap or an alcohol -based hand sanitizer. With soap, lather well, and then for at least thirty seconds longer wash between each finger and under the nails. Rinse thoroughly.

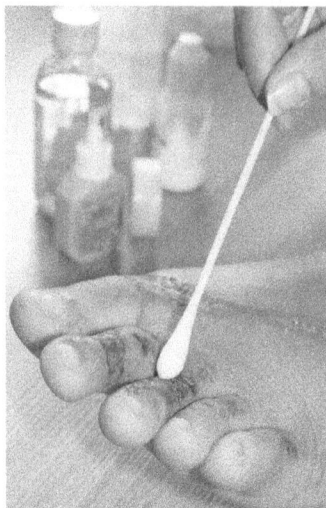

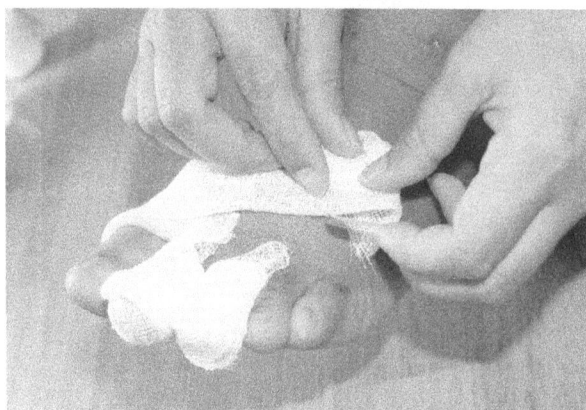

Cleansing and then dressing chronic toe ulcers

Surgeons scrub their hands for four to five minutes to disinfect them prior to operating.

The best way to cleanse a cut, scrape, or wound, whether acute or chronic, is to flush the area copiously (for three to five minutes) with clean tap water. This removes dirt, bacterial contamination, and debris. Normal saline solution can be used but is not necessary. Any comfortable temperature is fine although cool water usually feels better on burns. Kitchen sink sprayers and showers are excellent, and you can safely use mild soaps like Dove™ or Dial™ on all wound types (acute and chronic). Avoid soaps with fragrance, triclosan, or triclocarban as these can irritate tissue and inhibit healing.

If the wound is extremely dirty, *gently* scrub it with a clean washcloth or gauze. Carefully work contaminants back out the way they entered. Use light pressure; hard scrubbing may disrupt the area and prolong healing time without added benefit. If cleaning the wound thoroughly is unbearably painful, seek medical assistance for appropriate anesthesia and cleansing. If you cause minor bleeding during wound cleansing, then use direct pressure.

For proper cleaning, tap water or saline is best, as many commercial wound cleaners are somewhat toxic to cells in the wound bed. Pouring full-strength Betadine or hydrogen peroxide on a wound will not only kill bacteria but will also harm healthy tissue and inhibit healing.

---

2. Dressing Your Wound

After cleansing your wound, we recommend drying it by exposing it to natural sunlight. Limited sun exposure is healthy for wounds and the UV light can help activate the healing processes and reduce infection. It is important to avoid scabbing,

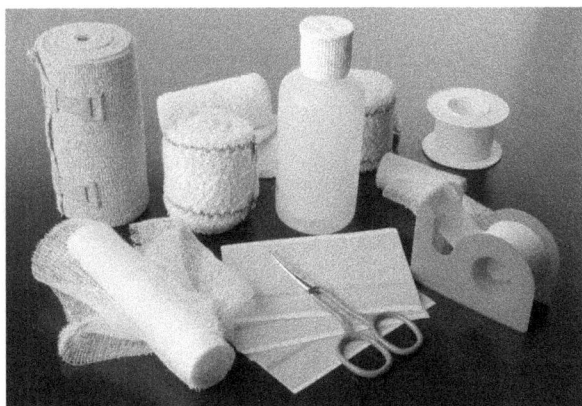

so we do not recommend prolonged exposure. Ten to fifteen minutes in the sun should be adequate. If sunlight is not available, pat it dry with a soft clean cloth.

After drying your wound, it is time for a dressing. Chapter 14 contains more detailed information on dressing types and materials. Dressings should maintain an optimal moist environment (prevents scabbing) and protect the wound from further damage and contamination. We recommend applying a topical ointment to help facilitate a moist and antiseptic environment. Small wounds can be covered with a large Band-Aid or similar product. For larger wounds, place clean (or sterile) dry gauze over the topical ointment. Some of the "non-adherent" products like Telfa™ are coated with plastic and do not absorb wound drainage well.

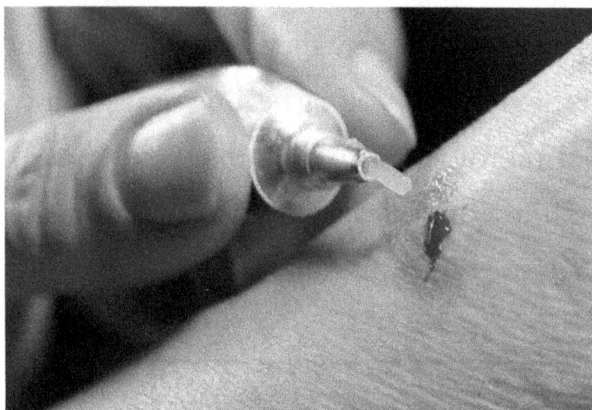

If the gauze eventually starts sticking to the wound, then moisten or rinse in a shower or under a sink sprayer and carefully remove it. Use more topical coating the next time or switch to Telfa. If the gauze becomes soaked with drainage from the wound, you may need to change it more frequently or seek an especially absorbent product such as an alginate or foam dressing.

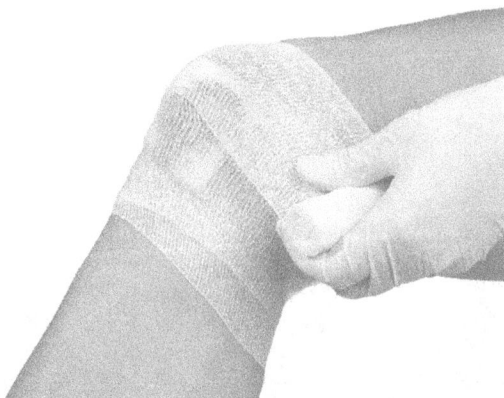

Tape can be used to secure dressings but will not stick well if there is a lot of drainage. Also, many people eventually develop reactions to the adhesives, and tape can damage fragile skin. A better alternative is roll gauze to hold the dressing in place. Tape the gauze to itself.

Regarding topical preparations, avoid antibiotic ointments containing neomycin; it commonly causes allergic and inflammatory reactions. Bacitracin is better tolerated. By far, our favorite over-the-counter product is medical grade honey (to be discussed). Coconut oil is another great option which has multiple benefits including maintaining a moist environment, facilitating fibroblast proliferation and eradicating both bacteria (*Staphylococcus aureus*) and fungi (*Candida albicans*). Sold as a cream, calendula is a potent medicinal herb derived from the marigold plant with antibacterial, antiviral, and anti-inflammatory properties.

3. Skin Tears

Skin tears are common in the elderly, especially on the hands, forearms, and legs. They can occur even with minor friction or shearing. Aging skin becomes thinner, drier, and less elastic, and therefore more fragile. They should be carefully rinsed and if there is skin folded back on itself, it should be gingerly brought back to cover the wound, one of the topical treatments applied, a non-adherent pad (this is a good time for Telfa pads if there is not a lot of drainage), and a light wrap should be applied.

Seek medical help if bleeding does not stop (especially if you take blood thinners), the wound goes any deeper than the skin, or has a thick flap (which could possibly benefit from sutures, glue, or steri-strips). When in doubt, get it checked out. For minor skin tears with minimal bleeding, transparent dressings (like Tegaderm®) can be left in place for three to five days. Wounds are still visible beneath these dressings.

II. CARING FOR A CHRONIC NON-HEALING WOUND

In addition to the recommendations already given, chronic problem wounds demand even more. As we previously discussed, wound centers focus on "off-loading," which means taking pressure off the wound. The more the wounded extremity is used, the more force, pressure, or friction on the wound, the less likely it is to heal quickly (or at all).

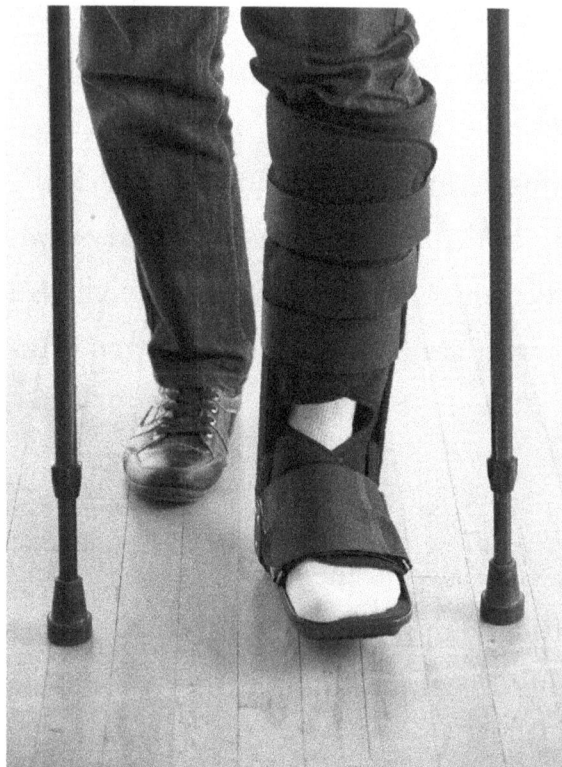

Walking cast to off-load pressure to bottom of foot

You would be surprised how much appropriate off-loading can help the healing process. Techniques vary depending on the wound location and include crutches, wheelchairs, knee scooters, walking casts, walking boots, wedge shoes, or open-toed shoes. These are certainly things you can do at home, and even if you cannot get a prescription for some of these, use common sense. For example, foam dressings help minimize pressure on a wound. Bottom line: try not to put any pressure or stress on the area with the wound; keeping pressure off may be the *only* way to heal completely.

In addition to off-loading with the purpose of eliminating excessive pressure, the term "surgical offloading" describes a surgeon correcting deformities of the foot or ankle to help spread the pressure about and decrease pressure on the wounded area. The obvious risk here is creating a new surgical wound in someone who has already demonstrated poor healing potential. Sometimes it is successful, sometimes not. "Solving" one problem might lead to a new one; for example, amputating an infected toe creates a much higher risk of wounds elsewhere in the foot due to increased pressure in another (compensatory) area.

If your wounds are the result of leg swelling because of poor venous circulation or a condition known as lymphedema (in which your lymphatic channels do not work well), then controlling edema with compression therapy is a critical step in healing. Sometimes wound physicians prescribe sophisticated compression pumps to help with veno-lymphatic disease or recommend custom-fit compression stockings or garments. It is important that your arterial function be evaluated prior to starting aggressive compression therapy, and if you have significant pain, discomfort, or discoloration of your toes, you should stop it immediately. If your leg swelling is

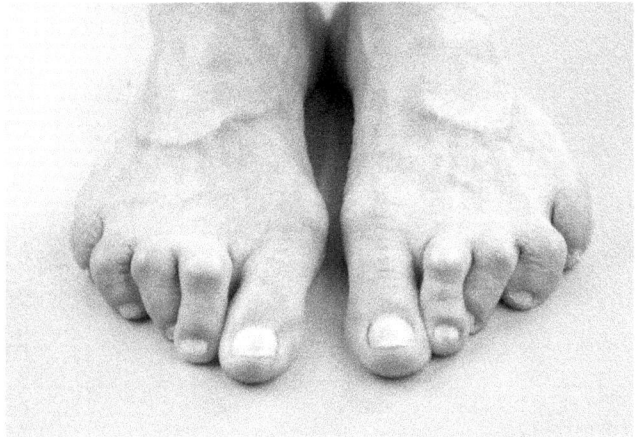

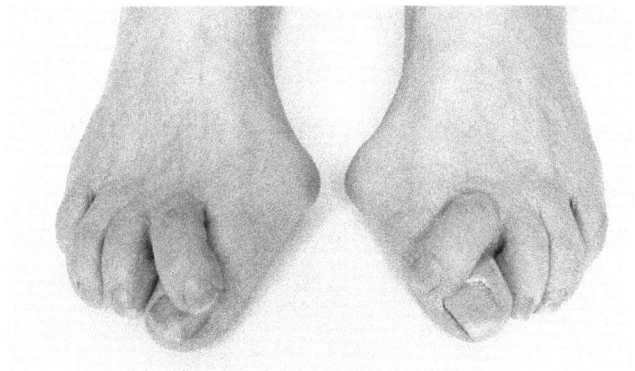

See any potential for pressure ulcers here?

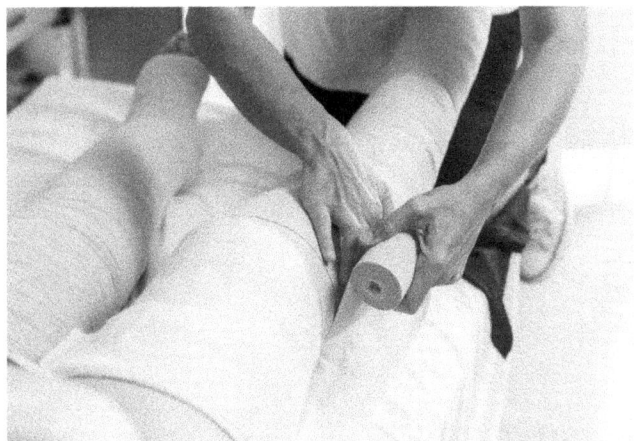

Application of a three-layer compression wrap at a wound care center

149

caused by congestive heart failure, you might benefit from diuretics ("water pills"), elevation, and gentle compression.

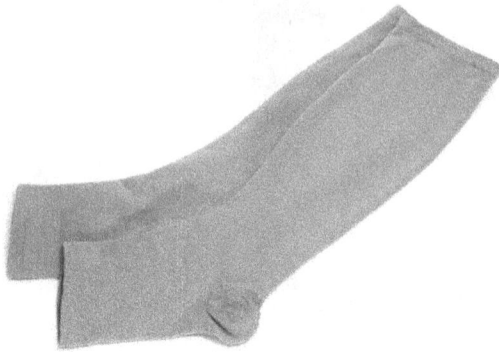

A useful alternative is commercially available over-the-counter compression stockings (one commonly found brand is "TED Hose"). Although perhaps not as effective as pumps and custom-fit garments, these stockings are readily available and can make a huge difference. Other measures to reduce lower extremity swelling include walking and exercising—muscle contractions help increase venous and lymphatic return. Also, keeping your legs elevated when possible helps. The less time sitting and standing the better. Wounds do not heal well in edematous areas.

CHAPTER 13

Heal with Steel

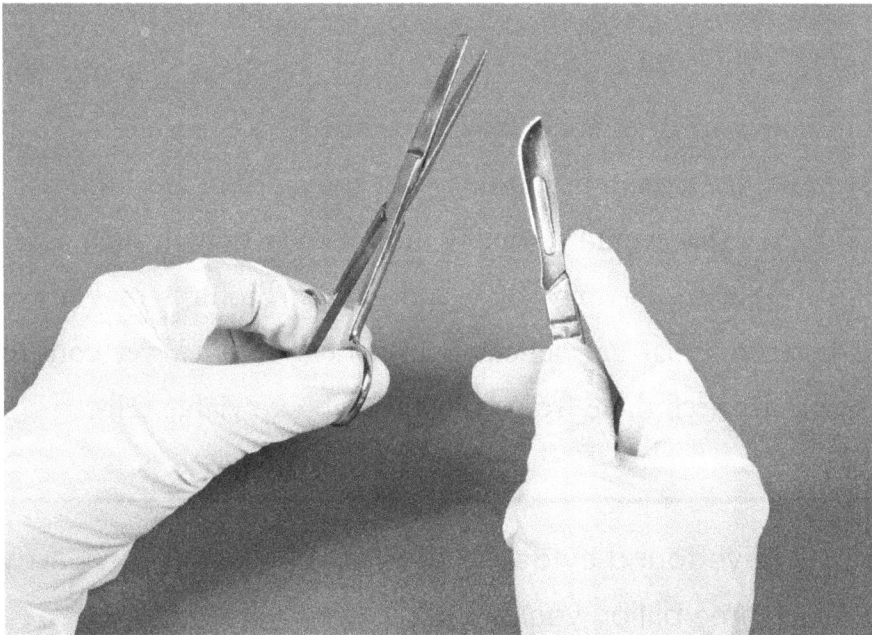

While healing your body from the inside, it is equally important to begin healing the wound on the outside. The wound base requires restoration in order to reconstruct healthy tissue. Dead tissue, debris, and biofilm must be destroyed and eliminated. The best way to accomplish this is debridement.

The primary cause of a recalcitrant wound is a chronic low-grade infection produced by a microscopic "biofilm," which keeps the wound stuck in the inflammatory phase. Biofilm is composed of bacterial colonies, cellular debris, and extracellular polymeric substances (almost like scaffolding, secreted by various cells including the bacteria) that do not allow white blood cells, antibodies, and other host (your body's) immune defenses to penetrate. It can form a firm layer called eschar. Systemic and even topical antibiotics are often ineffective and unable to penetrate.

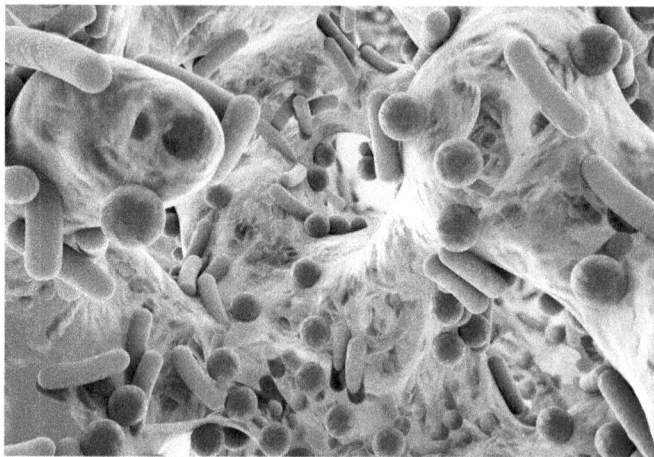

Biofilm of antibiotic resistant, rod-shaped and spherical bacteria (Escherichia coli, Pseudomonas aeruginosa, Klebsiella, MRSA)

Many of the bacteria in biofilm develop tolerance to antibiotics and environmental factors that would normally inhibit their growth such as UV light, pH changes, desiccation, osmolality, and others. Biofilms may also contain senescent host cells that are deficient in cellular activity, yet consume vital nutrients, thereby keep them from being available to viable cells.

Scientists have found evidence of biofilms existing on Earth for more than three billion years.

Effective debridement allows wounds stuck in the inflammatory phase to finally progress to the proliferative phase of healing. Ultimately, the single best treatment strategy for ridding a chronic wound of biofilm, and often the first essential step toward healing, is debridement.

1. SURGICAL DEBRIDEMENT

Sharp debridement (also known as surgical debridement) is one of the best reasons to go to a wound center. Weekly debridement of chronic ulcers helps them heal faster. Cardinal et al. showed that venous leg ulcers had a much more rapid reduction in size with sharp debridement versus no sharp debridement. In addition, wound centers that performed more frequent debridements had faster rates of wound closure.

Physicians may use a scalpel, a special tool called a curette, surgical scissors, or tissue nippers to debride wounds. They may excise only skin, slough, and debris; this is called a "selective" debridement. In other situations, it may be necessary to excise necrotic subcutaneous tissue, fat, muscle, tendon, and even bone. This type of deep debridement requires a detailed knowledge of both normal and pathologic anatomy, bleeding risk, adequate blood flow to the area, along with the right instruments, which have been properly sterilized. It takes a trained eye, considerable expertise, and careful technique to debride in a way that preserves the vital living and healing tissue, yet removes the devitalized tissue and infectious and dead material that is preventing the wound from healing appropriately.

In many cases, especially in patients with diabetic neuropathy and significant loss of sensation, debridement can be done without any anesthetic. However, some wounds require the use of topical or other anesthetic medications to make the procedure tolerable.

Even after sharp debridement, in a chronic wound, inflammatory processes can continue to generate microscopic cellular debris. Sometimes application of a topical enzymatic agent such as Collagenase SANTYL® is beneficial after debridement.

Case Report

Mrs. V is an eighty-two-year-old diabetic woman enjoying her backyard on a hot ninety-degree day. She decided to go inside and cool down but never made it. The last thing she remembers is feeling weak and dizzy. That evening when the daughter returned from work, she found Mrs. V unconscious—and very hot! Paramedics took her to the ER where she was found to have a body temperatureof 106 F and was admitted to the ICU with heat stroke.

After two days of cooling measures and rehydration, she finally regained full consciousness. She had developed large blisters from second-degree sunburns on both lower legs. At discharge, her granddaughter was instructed to dress the wounds with Bacitracin and gauze every day. While her granddaughter was away at work, Mrs. V, who had a bit of dementia, kept removing the bandages. The granddaughter was worried because the wounds were looking drier and darker, but she kept doing as she had been told.

Nearly a month after she had been discharged from the hospital, Mrs. V's legs became red, swollen, and very painful around the chronic wounds. She was taken to the ER, started on antibiotics, and referred to the wound center.

After assessing her vascular status, I debrided most of the black eschar and started daily application of Collagenase SANTYL®

ointment and moist gauze dressings. I explained the importance of keeping her dressings in place and recommended a special stocking to make removal of the dressings difficult. The following week, her wounds measured about the same, but I was now able to debride the rest of the eschar and nonviable tissue, which was now moist yellow and soft. I continued the SANTYL® one more week, and at her second follow-up visit, both wounds measured markedly smaller. Debridement was no longer painful, and she went on to heal completely after four more weekly visits.

The simple act of surgical debridement with appropriate topical care transformed her chronic wounds into actively healing wounds. Without it, especially at her age, the eschars would have eventually led to worsening infection, deeper wounds and tissue damage, and possibly even sepsis (overwhelming infection), or possibly death.

Although surgical debridement is a tremendous tool, there are exceptions: if you have a gangrenous wound or an arterial/ischemic ulcer, the arterial problem *must* be addressed first. There are also a few skin conditions where a sharp debridement can also make the ulcer worse. These include pyoderma gangrenosum, malignancy, or calciphylaxis. Your doctor must recognize these conditions and work with the appropriate specialist to treat the underlying condition before any type of debridement is undertaken. Biopsy of your wound might be recommended to ensure accurate diagnosis of your condition.

While debridement is a powerful technique for helping wounds heal, sharp debridement should not be done at home! Without the proper and appropriately sterilized tools, proper techniques, and, most importantly, the knowledge of which tissue and how much to remove, it is possible to cause more damage to a wound and make things worse. *This technique must be left to well-trained and experienced wound physicians.*

2. LASER DEBRIDEMENT

Laser debridement is a newer technology that ablates the wound bed to a precise depth and vaporizes biofilm. It can change the wound microbiota and the wound bed surface. It is much less commonly used than sharp debridement, and it is only currently FDA approved for pressure ulcers. However, other wound types, such as pyoderma gangrenosum, also benefit from the use of debridement lasers such as erbium lasers. As usual, insurance typically will not pay for off-label treatments such as these; therefore, they are not available at conventional wound centers.

3. NON-SURGICAL DEBRIDEMENT

Although skilled surgical debridement is the most effective way to control the biofilm of wounds, there is a variety of non-surgical debridement techniques—and some are suitable for home use.

We do not recommend at home use of wet-to-dry dressings. They can be very painful and also pull off or damage viable tissue. We also do not recommend using Betadine or hydrogen peroxide (which lead to tissue damage) or soaking your wound in Epsom salts (which leads to tissue desiccation).

Another debridement method described in the literature, although rarely used is "biological debridement" with medical grade maggots (we kid you not!). Up to you on this one—we think unless properly done (and how is that?) the hygiene and disgust factor absolutely precludes this method.

Gently scrubbing a wound with moistened gauze in the shower after soaking it and washing it well with mild soap as previously discussed is a form of mechanical debridement, which can be helpful. Keeping moist dressings on it to maintain the healing environment is usually helpful, unless the wound is draining copiously.

By far, our favorite methods of non-surgical debridement are enzymatic debridement and autolytic debridement. Both also help promote the all-important moist healing environment.

Enzymatic debridement with Collagenase SANTYL® ointment is an excellent way to reduce wound bioburden without harming healthy tissue and is often the best choice for a wound dressing until completely viable granulation tissue is established. Unfortunately, this excellent (and one of a kind) product is still not available over the counter, and because it is still under patent, it remains quite expensive. It is very safe but should not be used on third-degree burns or malignancies. Even if your doctor does not specialize in wound care, consider educating your doctor about it and asking for a prescription for it.

Finally, autolytic debridement with medical grade honey is one of the best, least expensive, and easily accessible over-the-counter methods to use on your wounds at home. See Chapter 14 for more on this wonderful product.

References and Recommended Reading

1. Cardinal M, Eisenbud DE, Armstrong DG, et al. "Serial surgical debridement: a retrospective study on clinical outcomes in chronic lower extremity wounds." *Wound Repair Regen*, 2009; 17: 306-311.

2. Warriner RA, Wilcox JR, Carter MJ, and Stewart DG. "More Frequent Visits to Wound Care Clinics Results in Faster Times to Close Diabetic Foot and Venous Leg Ulcers." *Adv Skin Wound Care*, 2012; 25 (11): 494-501.

3.   Wolcott, R. "Providing a Biofilm Explanation for Ablative Treatment of Recalcitrant Wounds." *Today's Wound Clinic*, Sept 2016; 12-18.

CHAPTER 14

Dressings: Pour Some Honey on That

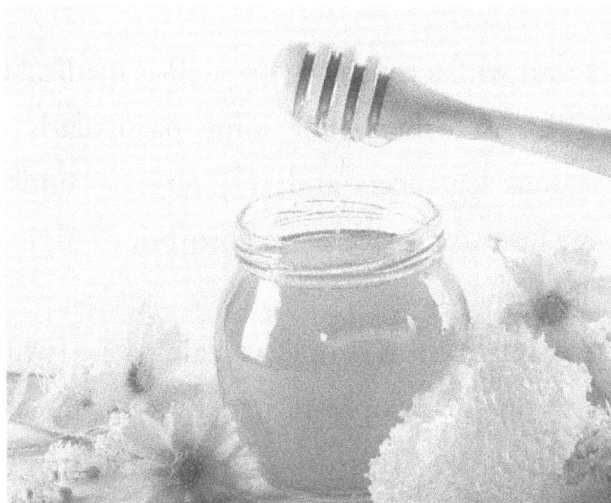

This chapter discusses types of dressings available to the consumer for purchase, some of which are used commonly in wound centers. The next chapter details dressings and other modalities that require prescriptions or a doctor's help to obtain.

DRESSINGS

After debridement, the next step is choosing the best dressing. Dressing selection can be confusing for patients (and doctors not trained in wound care). Understanding which dressing will make an immediate impact on the wound is important, and this may change weekly as the wound progresses.

First, let's define how we use the term "dressing." Although you may think of dressings as gauze, tape, and bandages, we think of a wound dressing as the combination of products, often in layers, that cover the wound. Dressings serve multiple functions including ensuring proper wound bed moisture (which may involve adding moisture to a dry wound or absorbing excess moisture from a draining wound), protecting the wound from further damage, treating infection, and removing foreign material. Some dressings facilitate passive debridement, antimicrobial agent delivery, and medication delivery. Additional factors to consider when choosing dressing materials include the necessary frequency of reapplication, cost, ability to perform at home, and availability.

Many dressings start with a topical agent such as medical honey, calendula, gentamicin, SANTYL®, or others. For some particularly heavily draining wounds (such as venous leg ulcers and very large wounds), an alginate or other layer may come next to provide extra absorption. Alginate, derived from seaweed, is one such substance.

The covering layer might be as simple as plain gauze (which is inexpensive and has good absorption) or a sophisticated product like highly absorptive foams or hydrofiber dressings. This dressing material may be held in place with tape, an elastic bandage, or gauze ("roll gauze"). The specific choices of roll gauze, tape, and elastic bandages are typically matters of cost, availability, comfort, and preference. In some cases, a special cast or off-loading boot may be the final step that helps take pressure off the wound. Although not technically part of the dressing, these can be very important for wound healing, particularly on the soles of the feet.

A list and brief description of some of the best dressing products we have found follows (listed in alphabetical order).

1. ALOE VERA

Aloe vera topical skin gel (0.5% or higher) is very effective for improving healing of acute and chronic wounds, burns, and frostbite. The mucilaginous gel acts on fibroblasts during tissue formation and stimulates collagen deposition. Aloe vera has anti-inflammatory and antifungal properties, and (when ingested) it has gastro-protective and blood-sugar-lowering effects.

2. CALENDULA

Calendula, derived from the marigold flower, has been used to cleanse wounds and promote healing for thousands of years. The ancient Egyptians prized it for its rejuvenating properties. At one time, the most common surgeries were amputations caused by infected wounds. An old British folk saying is *"Where there is calendula, there is no need of a surgeon."*

Calendula has a variety of beneficial properties for wound healing. It helps destroy bacteria, viruses, and fungi. It is a powerful anti-inflammatory and can help

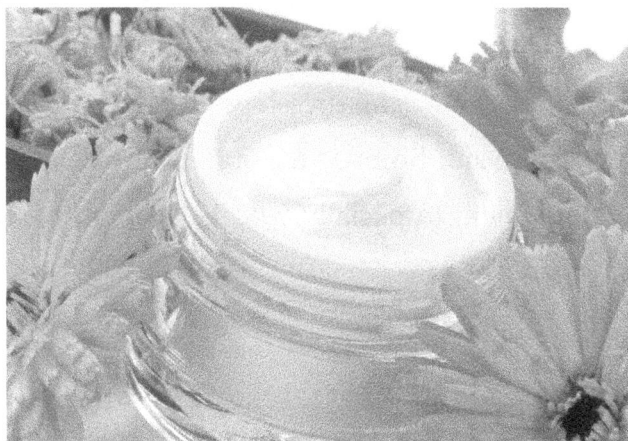

break the chronic inflammatory state of some wounds. It also promotes cellular growth and epithelialization.

Calendula (usually 2–10% concentration) is available in tinctures, ointments, creams, and washes. It can be applied to ulcers, burns, bruises, and cuts/lacerations. It also can be used for nosebleeds, varicose veins, hemorrhoids, rectal inflammation (proctitis), inflammation of the eyelids, rashes, itching, acne, and eczema.

3. COCONUT OIL

Coconut oil has antioxidant, anti-inflammatory, and antimicrobial properties. It helps repair the gut and improves immune function. Used topically on wounds, its benefits include strengthening epidermal tissue and removing dead skin cells (passive debridement) for superficial wounds. Coconut oil protects against sunburn and is excellent for many chronic skin conditions including atopic dermatitis (eczema).

4. COLLAGEN DRESSINGS

Collagen is a critical structural protein in skin that gives tensile strength. Collagen dressings (Promogran® is a good example) provide binding sites for healing proteins in the wound bed. It comes in powder, gel, and solid forms. Combination dressings also exist which combine collagen with alginate (Colactive and Epiona are good examples). Collagen can also be taken orally as a supplement (especially type 1 collagen) to further improve healing.

5. ESSENTIAL OILS

- **Frankincense oil** has astringent properties that help decrease bleeding and speed healing. It promotes cellular regeneration and is excellent for treating dry skin and reducing scarring.

- **Myrrh oil**, found in creams and lotions, has been valued since ancient Egyptian times for its wound-healing and infection-fighting properties.

- **Olive leaf extract** is a popular folk remedy from Turkey. It has powerful anti-inflammatory properties and helps increase immune system function. It can be used orally or topically on wounds.

- **Argan oil**, used for generations in Morocco, is rich in vitamins A and E, omega-6 fatty acids, and linoleic acid. It works well on wounds, acne, bug bites, eczema, psoriasis, and helps moisturize skin so it looks and feels youthful.

- **Geranium oil** has antiseptic properties that ward off bacterial infections. It also speeds healing of acute wounds by enhancing hemostasis (blood clotting) and, in doing so, helps prevent toxins from reaching your bloodstream through the open wound. It has been used to treat eczema, fungal infections including athlete's foot, burns, frostbite, and general itching.

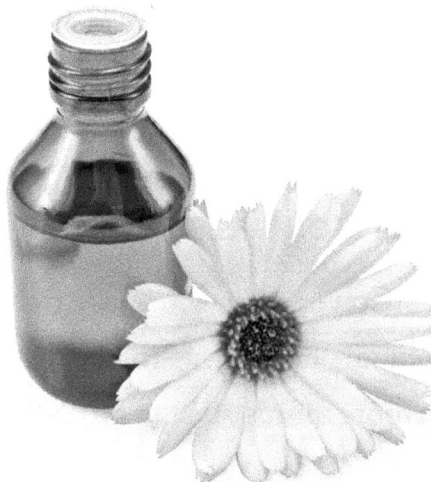

- **Persian oak** is a traditional Iranian remedy with polyphenolic components that speed up wound contracture (decreasing the size of the wound) and thus wound healing.

- **Tea tree oil** (*Melaleuca alternifolia*) has been used for hundreds of years in Australia for skin care and to naturally fight acne. Like many of the essential oils, it has potent antimicrobial and anti-inflammatory properties.

6. HEMCON DRESSINGS

HemCon bandages are made from a protein (chitosan) found in shrimp, which promotes hemostasis (blood clotting) and offers antibacterial action against microorganisms such as MRSA and VRE—two common antibiotic-resistant pathogens. It is excellent to stop bleeding and adheres well to wounds.

7. HONEY

Honey has been used as a wound dressing for thousands of years. Manuka honey from New Zealand has been proven so effective that it has recently been FDA approved for wound care in the United States. This honey is produced by bees foraging on the flowers of the medicinal Manuka bush, and it is a potent broad-spectrum antimicrobial agent that may be more effective than conventional antibiotics against some forms of bacteria, including even the dreaded Methicillin Resistant Staph aureus (MRSA). In addition, bacteria do not appear to be able to develop resistance. Additional beneficial properties of honey for wound healing include:

1. Promoting a slightly acidic wound environment, which increases oxygen release from hemoglobin, and makes the wound bed inhospitable to many bacteria.

2. The high osmolarity of honey draws fluid out of the wound bed to create an outflow of lymph. Like a miniature wound vac, this draws the tissue together and promotes wound contraction.

3. The high sugar content desiccates and inhibits the growth of bacteria.

4. Glucose oxidase, an enzyme from honey, releases therapeutic levels of hydrogen peroxide into the wound bed.

5. Honey performs autolytic debridement of nonviable tissue and performs autolytic debridement of nonviable tissue, which helps eliminate established biofilms and prevents formation of new ones.

Unfortunately, the standard highly processed "Grade A" honey (in a bear shaped dispenser) available at your local grocer is not the right stuff. Many commercially available honey products are pasteurized (which destroys some of the beneficial properties) and contain added sweeteners, including the most evil of them all—high-fructose corn syrup. HFCS is likely to *increase* infection and should never ever be used on wounds.

Locally sourced organic raw honey can be used on your wounds but likely does not have the demonstrated potency of New Zealand Manuka honey. Manuka honey has a variety of benefits when eaten also, including stimulating the immune system and healing the gut.

Manuka honey products are commercially available, including the excellent MediHoney® products. You can buy these as topical gels, pastes, or honey impregnated dressings. Use honey on lacerations, abrasions, cuts, scalds/burns, sunburns, and post-operative incision sites, and of course chronic and non-healing wounds. The only contraindications (reasons not to use) honey-based dressings on your wounds are third-degree burns (you should be treated by a burn center for those anyway), malignancy, or allergy to honey products.

If it's not clear—we love honey dressings! It is also great for veterinary wounds because if an animal licks off the dressing, honey is completely safe when ingested. We recently used MediHoney® gel to heal our pet turtle's injured shell; it cured our guinea pig's ringworm and worked great on our dog's cut from barbed-wire.

8. HYDROCOLLOID DRESSINGS

Hydrocolloid dressings are flexible, absorbent dressings made from a gel-like substance that is excellent for maintaining an optimal moist healing environment and protecting wounds from further contamination and trauma. They usually stick to periwound skin without tape or cover bandages. They are particularly effective for eliminating the pain of burns. They are excellent for wounds over bony prominences—such as the ankle. They are not particularly absorptive and so should not be used on blisters or heavily draining wounds. They do not have intrinsic antimicrobial activity so should be used with care or combined with an antimicrobial dressing in wounds where infection is present or suspected, such as diabetic foot ulcers. A commonly used brand is DuoDERM®.

One of our new favorite combination dressings is a honey-impregnated hydrocolloid. It can be left on a wound for up to a week and is waterproof so you can shower with it. The combination of wound protection, moist healing, and convenience of the hydrocolloid, paired with the healing properties of honey, make this a great choice for dry wounds.

9. IODINE IMPREGNATED DRESSINGS

Although pouring iodine or Betadine onto a wound can be detrimental to healing, there are a number of dressings available that provide a safe way to use the powerful disinfectant properties of iodine for chronic wounds. Iodosorb® and Iodoflex® are cadexomer iodine-based wound dressings which have been shown to be effective at controlling infection and reducing biofilm. Iodine dressings are particularly useful for a limited time period on infected diabetic foot ulcers or foul-smelling wounds.

10. METHYL-GENTIAN DRESSINGS

Excellent antimicrobial combination dressing can be created by pairing the antibacterial properties of methylene blue with the antifungal properties of gentian violet. An example of this is Hydrofera BLUE®. These dressings are useful on a broad range of infected wounds including diabetic ulcers and venous leg ulcers. Hydrofera BLUE® Flex is a soft, moldable, absorbent foam that works great over pressure ulcers, bony prominences, and under compression wraps.

11. PHMB

Polyhexamethylene biguanide (PHMB) has been used for over sixty years as an antimicrobial agent. It is a positively charged substance that binds to negatively charged bacterial cell membranes. This disrupts and weakens the cell membrane, rendering microbes impotent. Dressings with PHMB help to prevent the reformation of biofilm in chronic wounds (which typically occurs two to three days or less after debridement).

12. SILVER

Hippocrates first described the antimicrobial properties of silver in 400 BC. During World War I, soldiers used silver to treat infected wounds. Dilute silver eyedrops are used in newborn babies to prevent conjunctivitis. The antibacterial action of silver is dependent on the silver ion. It works by destabilizing bacterial cell membranes, making them more porous (thus potentiating the action of other antibiotics). It also interferes with bacterial metabolism, forcing the production of lethal toxic metabolites.

Commercial wound dressings usually pair silver with collagen, alginate, or foam. Silver nanoparticles have also been incorporated into excellent wound gels. The antibacterial action of silver dressings is further enhanced by the presence of an electric field. (More about this in our microcurrent section, Chapter 18.)

SO WHAT SHOULD YOU USE?

Given all the great options, you may wonder how to choose the best dressing for your wound. Experienced wound care clinicians go through complex decision trees in order to make this choice, but we will try to give you a few guidelines. First, *you cannot go wrong with a Manuka honey product.* It is anti-inflammatory and antimicrobial and facilitates autolytic debridement and maintains a moist healing environment. It is inexpensive and widely available. It is non-toxic, effective, and safe to start using on any wound. It is also great for ingrown toenails and cold sores. A lot of fake manuka honey (some adulterated with syrup) is being sold (both in stores and on Amazon). They do not have the same anti-microbial activity or effectiveness as real manuka honey, so beware.

The next issue is moisture control. If you have a dry wound, then application of a Manuka honey product topped with dry gauze or one of the honey hydrocolloid dressings may be all you need. If you have a damp, draining, or moist wound, or if your dressings start to get damp or moist with wound exudate, then you will need to change the dressings more often or use an absorptive substance over the top of the honey or honey alginate. Removing excess drainage and moisture from the wound bed is important for biofilm control and skin protection. Sometimes using a highly absorbent foam cover is also necessary.

Using a dressing type which is too absorbent can dry the wound prematurely. Realize that as a wound heals, it goes through different stages and may require a different dressing type for each stage. With careful observation, you will begin to understand how to find the right balance.

Obviously, as you are going through this process, it is important to closely monitor the progress of your wound. If your wound seems to be worsening, then we recommend you seek qualified help from a physician experienced in wound care. We actually recommend that anyway.

References and Recommended Reading

1. Chithra P, Sajithlal BG. Chandrakasan G. "Influence of Aloe vera on the healing of dermal wounds in diabetic rats." *J Ethnopharmacol.* 1998; 59(3):195-201.

2. Reynolds T, Dweck AC. "Aloe vera leaf gel: a review update." *J Ethnopharmacol.* 1999; 68 (1): 3-37.

3. Rao SG, et al. "Calendula and Hypericum: two homeopathic drugs promoting wound healing in rats." *Fitoterapia.* 1991; 62 (6): 508-10.

4. Leach M. "Calendula officinalis and Wound Healing: A Systematic Review." *WOUNDS* 2008; 20 (8).

5. Lavasanijou MR, et al. "Wound Healing Effects of Quercus Brantii and Pelargonium Graveolens Extracts in Male Wistar Rats." WOUNDS 2016; 28 (10): 369-375.

6. Majno, Guido. *The Healing Hand: Man and Wound in the Ancient World.* New York, NY: Classics of Medicine Library, 1991. Print.

7. Mercola, Joseph. "What Are the Health Benefits of Coconut Oil?" *Mercola.com.* Dr. Mercola, 30 May 2016. Web. 11 June 2017.

8. Molan P, Rhodes T. "Honey: A Biologic Wound Dressing." *WOUNDS* 2015; 27 (6): 141-151.

9. www.dermasciences.com

10. Blair, S.E., Cokcetin, N.N., Harry, E.J. et al. "The unusual antibacterial activity of medical-grade *Leptospermum* honey: antibacterial spectrum, resistance and transcriptome analysis." *Eur J Clin Microbiol Infect Dis* (2009) 28: 1199.

11. Cooper, R.A., Jenkins, L., Henriques, A.F.M. et al. "Absence of bacterial resistance to medical-grade Manuka honey.*" Eur J Clin Microbiol Infect Dis* (2010) 29: 1237.

12. Lu, Jing et al. "Manuka-Type Honeys Can Eradicate Biofilms Produced by *Staphylococcus Aureus* Strains with Different Biofilm-Forming Abilities." Ed. Siouxsie Wiles. *PeerJ* 2 (2014): e326. *PMC.* Web. 12 June 2017.

13. Carson CF, Hammer KA, Riley TV. "Melaleuca alternifolia (Tea Tree) Oil: a Review of Antimicrobial and Other Medicinal Properties." *Clin Microbiol Rev.* 2006; 19(1): 50–62.

14. Waycaster C, Milne C. "Economic and Clinical Benefit of Collagenase Ointment Compared to a Hydrogel dressing for Pressure Ulcer Debridement in a Long-Term Care Setting." *WOUNDS* 2013; 25 (6): 141-147.

CHAPTER 15

Even More Hope for Healing

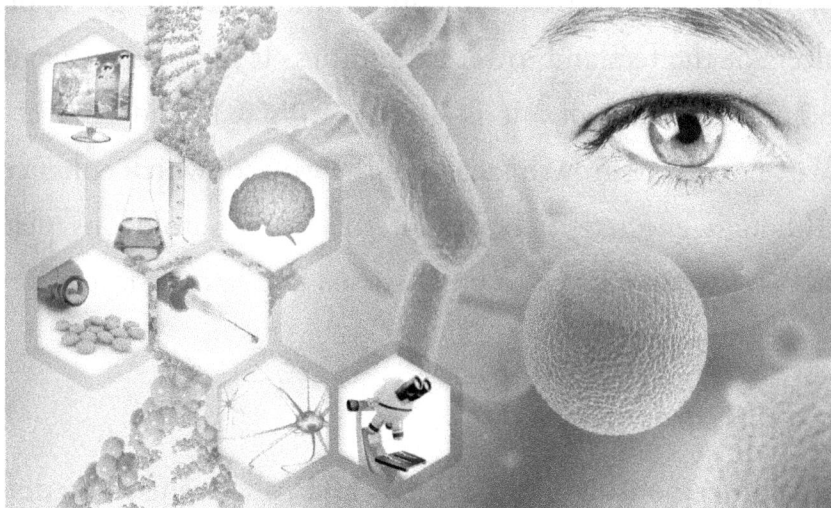

TOPICAL THERAPIES

1. Collagenase SANTYL Ointment

As previously discussed, Collagenase SANTYL® is the only enzymatic debridement agent currently available, an excellent choice for any wound with lots of dead tissue, such as chronic ulcers and severely burned skin. It enzymatically debrides nonliving tissue from wounds and destroys biofilm. It is still on patent and only available by prescription, so it can be quite expensive. It can effectively start the debridement process before you ever get to a wound center.

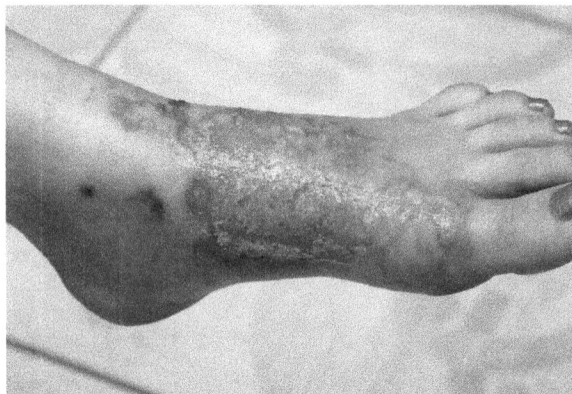

SANTYL helps debride a painful foot burn

We recommend asking your doctor for a prescription for SANTYL. Apply a two-millimeter-thick layer daily after cleansing with saline and then cover the wound with gauze.

2. Regranex

Regranex is an FDA-approved prescription-only wound gel approved for diabetic ulcers of the feet and lower extremities. It requires refrigeration and should be applied once daily. It is derived from Clostridium bacteria and provides platelet-derived growth factors to the wound, which enhances wound healing. Although effective, a better alternative is autologous platelet rich plasma (PRP) or even PRP gel, to be discussed in a later chapter.

3. Sulfonated Hydrocarbons

Sulfonated hydrocarbons (a brand name is HybenX) are used by dentists and approved by the FDA as a root canal cleanser. Similar to how it removes plaque from teeth, the sulfuric acid removes biofilm from wounds. Hydrocarbons are also known for eliminating odor. This liquid can be applied to complex wounds and can reach into crevices and deep, cavernous wounds such as pressure ulcers. Sulfonated hydrocarbons should be applied by experienced physicians; otherwise healthy tissue may be damaged. When combined with debridement, this therapy has helped many chronic recalcitrant wounds with biofilm finally progress to healing.

4. Topical Insulin

Recent research on both rats and human skin cells in culture has shown the wound healing benefits of insulin. This hormone, important for regulating blood sugar levels, can speed up the healing process when applied directly to a wound. How?

Insulin switches on cellular signaling proteins. This causes microvascular endothelial cells to migrate into the wound tissue and form new blood vessels. It also stimulates keratinocytes, the cells that regenerate the epidermis. This partially explains why diabetes correlates with poor healing.

Mix a few units of insulin with a few milliliters of saline and spread it on the wound. Topical insulin is very safe, especially in small doses, with virtually no side effects—it will not cause unsafe drops in blood sugar. Eventually there may be an insulin-based wound product, but you can certainly consider applying some insulin-saline solution to speed up the healing.

5. Testosterone Cream or Gel

Some data and our experience suggest that topical testosterone can be applied to a wound with great results. This usually involves partnering with a compound pharmacist to compound it into a water-based gel for best results.

6. T3 Thyroid Cream

There have been some studies showing that topical thyroid cream can benefit wound healing. We sometimes use this with patients who are still not healing well despite other measures.

7. Vitamin D Topical

You know all about the benefits of vitamin D, so is it any surprise that it might benefit wounds when applied topically? The synthetic vitamin-D analog is calcipotriene cream 0.005%, and it helps regulate skin cell production and development. It is approved for the treatment of psoriasis and porokeratosis, and it is another effective treatment for some wounds. Of course, the best source of vitamin D is in the sky during the daytime.

OTHER SPECIALIZED THERAPIES

1. "Smart" Dressings

Newer "smart" dressings are using nanotechnology by incorporating miniature electrical sensors into the dressing. These dressings are engineered to detect changes in a wound environment. They then alert the patient or doctor by altering the color of the dressing or sending a message to a smartphone. The doctor can then instruct the patient to change the dressing via a text message. They sound interesting … but we are concerned about the potential electromagnetic field (EMF) exposure of wearing such products continuously.

Certain bio-cellulose dressings have been developed which deliver topical antibiotics such as vancomycin. This makes sense, especially if it could eliminate the need for taking antibiotics, even in just a few cases. Soon, we may even be incorporating biologic material—such as stem cells—into dressings.

An international team of researchers has developed silver ion-coated scaffolds to hold (fat-derived adult) stem cells, which slow the spread of or kill MRSA while regenerating new bone. This provides a new potential treatment of osteomyelitis—without surgery.

Among other novel drugs and devices, a 3D inkjet printer has being developed for skin tissue engineering, and a gene-activated matrix has been developed for bone regeneration.

2. Pneumatic Compression Therapy

Patients with venous insufficiency and lymphedema sometimes only heal their wounds after adding pneumatic medicine. This means delivering peristaltic pulse pneumatic waveforms to the arms or legs. So-called "dynamic compression" helps stimulate normal circulation and lymphatic flow which has been lost.

Pneumatic compression devices are especially beneficial for patients with lymphedema, including cancer-related lymphedema. How does it work? While sitting at home, the device inflates over swollen areas of the limb or trunk to help move excess fluid out of the area. One study showed a dramatic 75 percent fewer episodes of cellulitis in lymphedema patients who used this device.

Case Report

Mrs. B is a sixty-five-year-old female with lower extremity venous infufficiency and multiple ulcers on both legs. Her wounds have been present for years. She has had three prior episodes of cellulitis requiring hospitalization for IV antibiotics. Previously tried treatments included wound dressings, elevation, exercise, compression stockings, ace-wrapping, bandaging, diuretics, debridement, and participation in a formal wound care program. After three weeks of daily home pneumatic medicine treatment that we ordered, she healed the last of her ulcers. She continues to treat her legs for one hour a day to keep the swelling down and prevent new wounds. She can also walk farther and faster now than before, since her legs are so much lighter.

These are devices available for independent home use that are very simple to set up and use. We program and electronically lock in an individualized compression prescription, leaving you nothing to worry about. That way, inappropriate pressures and gradients cannot inadvertently be programmed.

3. Biologics or "Skin Substitutes"

Most wound care center protocols advocate the use of "advanced" therapies after four or more weeks of failed standard wound care due to poorly healing wounds. We refer to these as "biologics" or "living cell therapies." There are almost countless such products on the market, including dehydrated amniotic membrane allografts (Amnioexcel, Amniomatrix, Epifix, NuShield, Neox, etc.), umbilical cord and amniotic membrane allograft (NeoxCord), living cell amniotic membrane allograft (Grafix), human fibroblast-derived dermal substitutes (Apligraf and Dermagraft), human acellular dermal matrix (Graftjacket and DermACELL), human skin products (Theraskin), and by the time of publication, there will likely be three or four more. Of this list, only Apligraf, Dermagraft, and Grafix are living cell-based therapies; the others are acellular but may act as a scaffold that allows the body to convert the matrix into functional tissue in wound repair.

Using these products prior to the wound bed being properly prepared is ineffective and wasteful. That is not to say that advanced biologics should not be utilized by trained wound experts. On the contrary, if they help a wound heal more quickly, everyone wins. The patient has less risk of developing a complication such as infection and avoids hospitalization or an amputation, or more quickly gets his or her life back. The cost of healing that wound is reduced compared to the cost of more clinic visits, dressing supplies, home nursing visits, etc. Unfortunately, however, not everyone has even the baseline health to heal *with* these advanced therapies.

4. Scar Treatment

Most people develop a scar because of having had surgery, a burn, or a chronic wound. Scars can cause functional, aesthetic, and psychological problems. Because of contracture, scar tissue constricts and decreases mobility. Many burn victims may have restricted use of their limbs or neck even after they are finally healed.

There are scar treatments (beyond topical creams) that now include cryotherapy, laser therapy, microneedling, and microcurrent. Cryotherapy is the use of very cold temperatures to reduce scarring. Lasers also have been used for this purpose for about ten years. Fractionated CO_2 lasers release the tension on scars. The newest laser rejuvenation procedures, such as CO_2 laser skin resurfacing and YAG (Yttrium-aluminum-garnet) laser surgery, combined with intense pulsed light, can help revise scar tissue into normal skin to improve mobility and function.

5. Cryotherapy

Wim Hof (the "Ice Man") has shown us that exposure to extreme cold is good for one's health, but unfortunately not many of us have the fortitude to immerse ourselves in an ice bath for an extended period. An electrically cooled whole body cryotherapy chamber is the next best thing. Cryotherapy helps with inflammatory disorders and pain, causes endorphin release, and benefits your overall health. Wounds should be kept covered though in the chamber. The chamber is cooled to approximately -142 degrees F, and most treatments last two and a half to three minutes. The goal is to achieve a skin temperature drop (measured with infrared before and right after treatment) of between thirty and forty-five degrees. The health benefits are multiple. Go to www. USCryotherapy.com to see if there is a center near you.

References and Recommended Reading

1. Sossamon, Jeff. "Silver ion coated medical devices could fight MRSA while creating new bone." *MU News Bureau Atom.* University of Missouri, 8 Feb. 2017. Web. 11 June 2017.

2. Mohiti-Asli M, Molina C, et al. "Evaluation of Silver Ion-Releasing Scaffolds in a 3D Coculture System of MRSA and Human Adipose-Derived Stem Cells for Their Potential Use in Treatment or Prevention of Osteomyelitis." *Tissue Eng Part A.* 2016 Nov;22(21-22):1258-1263.

3. Karaca-Mandic, Pinar, Alan T. Hirsch, Stanley G. Rockson, and Sheila H. Ridner. "The Cutaneous, Net Clinical, and Health Economic Benefits of Advanced Pneumatic Compression Devices in Patients With Lymphedema." *JAMA Dermatology* 151.11 (2015): 1187. Web.

4. Alvarez OM et al. "Effect of High-pressure, Intermittent Pneumatic Compression for the Treatment of Peripheral Arterial Disease and Critical Limb Ischemia in Patients Without a Surgical Option." *WOUNDS* 2015; 27 (11): 293-301.

5. "New Diagnostic Devices Offers Promise for Improved Wound Healing." *Advanced Tissue.* Advanced Tissue, 23 Aug. 2016. Web. 11 June 2017.

6. "Cryotherapy Treatment." *US Cryotherapy.* US Cryotherapy. Web. 11 June 2017.

7. www.icemanwimhof.com

CHAPTER 16

Infected or Not?

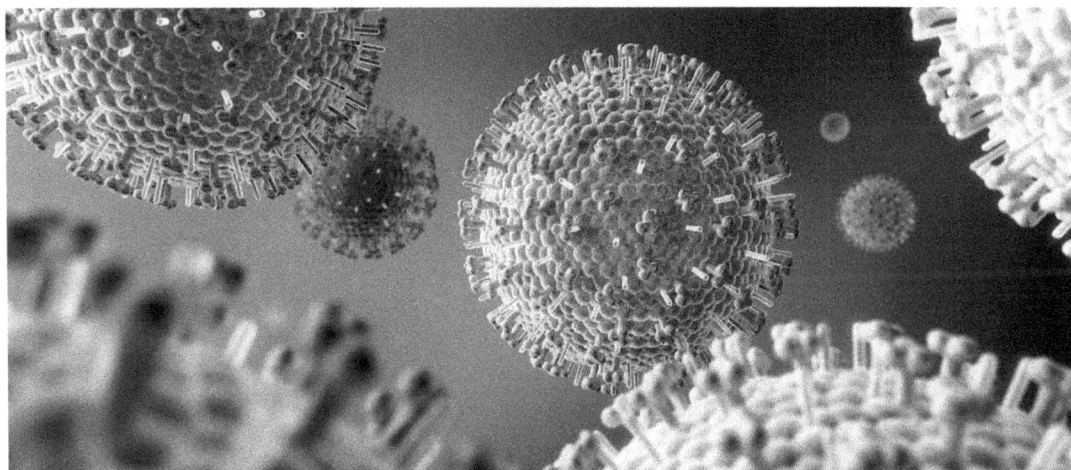

Bacteria are ubiquitous in the environment and on our skin. All chronic wounds contain bacteria. The degree of bacterial occupation of a wound is typically described as one of the following:

1. Contaminated wound: Surface bacteria are present, no detrimental impact upon healing. In fact, low levels of bacteria may actually

be beneficial by stimulating local white blood cells and proteolytic enzymes.

2. Colonized wound: Number of bacteria now competes with the host for local metabolic resources within the wound. This can be detrimental to healing.

3. Infected wound: Bacteria have reached a critical number, which arrests or reverses the healing process due to local tissue invasion and damage. This can spread, worsen, and become limb- or life-threatening.

An estimated 90 percent of chronic wounds are covered in a layer of physically adherent, interrelated microorganisms, which produce and maintain a polymeric substance matrix known as biofilm. This is at the very least colonization and at worst significant infection.

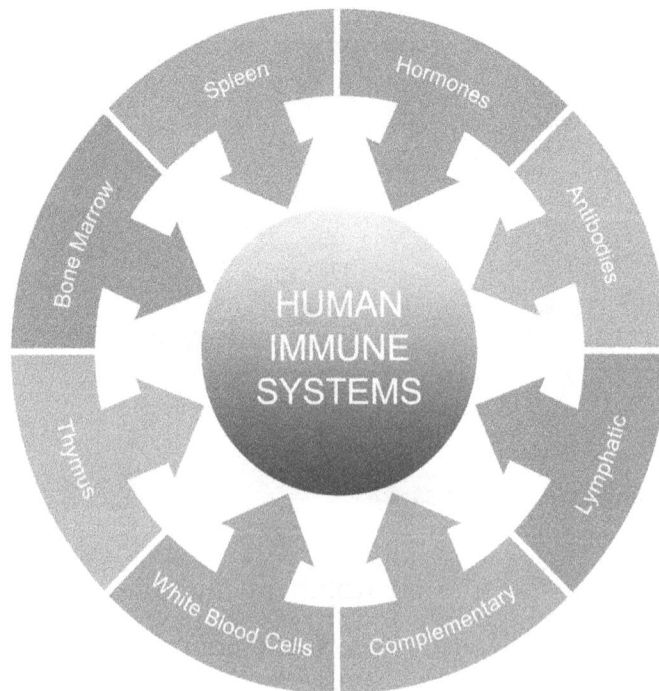

Our immune system is comprised of many systems, all of which affect our ability to resist infection

DEBRIDEMENT IS THE SOLUTION

The best way to manage biofilm is debridement, either active (surgical/sharp/mechanical) or passive (enzymatic/autolytic). Although antibiotics are frequently prescribed for chronic wounds, they are not effective at removing or eliminating the biofilm. One of the most common causes of non-healing wounds is poor blood flow, so the first problem with systemic antibiotics, given either intravenously or orally, is that the bloodstream may not carry them close to the site of the wound well.

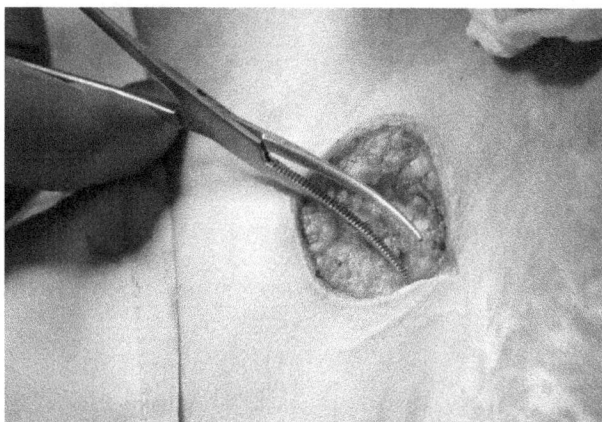

Even with adequate circulation and antibiotic delivery to the wound area, the antibiotic likely will not diffuse into the biofilm layer (which has no blood vessels), thus bacteria deep in the biofilm remain untouched by the antibiotic. Antibiotics typically only kill or injure growing and dividing bacteria. Some of the bacteria in the biofilm are dormant and therefore unaffected by antibiotics even if the medication gets to them. And of course, the more antibiotics floating around the environment the more likely bacteria with a variety of resistance mechanisms are selected for. This is certainly a problem with global implications but also can become distressingly personal for patients who are infected with bacteria for which there is no effective antibiotic.

In most cases, the use of a topical agent (silver, honey, methylene blue, calendula, iodine, etc.) in conjunction with appropriate biofilm disruption/debridement will be a better solution for treating the bacterial infection of wounds. Mechanically (or surgically) removing as much infected material as possible, followed by application of the antibiotic directly to the area of the infection, usually results in a higher local tissue concentration and thus more efficacy than one gets by the ingestion of antibiotic pills—and without the systemic side effects to the gut, etc.

POTENTIAL HARM FROM ANTIBIOTICS

In addition to the antibiotic resistance issue, antibiotics can cause real harm. Aside from the issue of repeated exposures potentially causing the development of allergies, many antibiotics have significant side effects like kidney damage and ototoxicity. Not only that, but as discussed, they disrupt gut flora, which can predispose you to virtually *any* disease. In some cases, by wiping out the "good" bacteria in the gut they allow the overgrowth of a potentially harmful species called *Clostridium difficile*, which can cause severe infections and even death.

Another example of potential harms, a popular class of antibiotics called fluoroquinolones (including ciprofloxacin and levofloxacin), just had an FDA "Black Box" warning issued against the first-line use of these medications. Part of the chemical structure of these antibiotics includes fluoride atoms, and as we have already discussed, fluoride can be toxic. It decreases the dielectric constant of water in exclusion zones in the body (effectively causing a "short-circuit") and can have serious detrimental bio-energetic effects.

Thousands worldwide have developed significant toxicities and side effects including orthopedic problems (tendonitis and even tendon rupture) and neurologic problems (neuropathy and other neurotoxicity) from quinolone antibiotics. Ironically, these medications have been touted for years as a first-line drug for most respiratory and urinary tract infections and were even required by the Centers for Medicare and Medicaid Services (CMS) Core Measures for the treatment of pneumonia, and doctors have been reprimanded for not prescribing them. This is not to say that there is never a place for quinolone antibiotics, just that your doctor needs to very carefully weigh the various risks and benefits, and if there is any other alternative it ought to be considered first.

WHEN ARE ANTIBIOTICS APPROPRIATE?

It is clear that disrupting and eliminating the biofilm is the most important principle in treating infected chronic wounds. The risks and problems with indiscriminate systemic antibiotic use are real, but that does not mean there is no place for antibiotics in treating your wound, just that they should be prescribed by a physician familiar with the care of non-healing wounds and used in conjunction with other therapies.

When prescribing antibiotics, your physician must carefully consider a number of factors including the wound type and severity, tissue perfusion (blood flow), the identity and virulence of the infecting organism, and the state of your immune system. Some organisms such as clostridial species, beta hemolytic streptococcus, and mycobacteria are especially likely to invade and cause tissue injury, and really do warrant aggressive antibiotic therapy.

If an infection is rapidly spreading or has become systemic in nature (sepsis) then immediate broad-spectrum antibiotic coverage may be necessary. However, the nature of chronic wounds is such that most of the time it is reasonable to wait for culture results to return so that your physician knows exactly what the primary infecting organism is and can select the best antibiotic tailored to eradicate that organism.

Wound cultures must be done carefully by knowledgeable personnel. Just swabbing the wound will lead to inaccurate and contaminated wound cultures. Obtaining a culture using this technique often reveals many bacterial species that may or may not be involved in creating the true pathology and, in fact, may not reveal the primary infecting agent. The wound should first be expertly debrided and then a deep culture obtained. Sometimes a tissue or bone biopsy is needed.

Recently, point-of-care biosensors designed to detect the presence of bacteria or proteins and enzymes that indicate wound infection have become available. Doctors drop a small amount of wound fluid onto the sensor, and the results are available in minutes. This can be done with each dressing change in order to monitor the progress of anti-infective treatment. A new and exciting auto-fluorescent detector technology ("bacteria-detecting camera") is being developed which will allow doctors to identify the culprit bacteria in real time, rather than waiting two to three days (or more) for the culture results. There are exciting changes coming!

Deciding when and which antibiotics are appropriate for non-healing wounds are often complicated decisions best left to physicians who specialize in wound care. Bone infections (osteomyelitis) require the most aggressive antibiotic therapy. Exposed surgical hardware with surrounding infection usually requires removal of the hardware since antibiotics cannot "sterilize" the wound with bacteria attached to hardware.

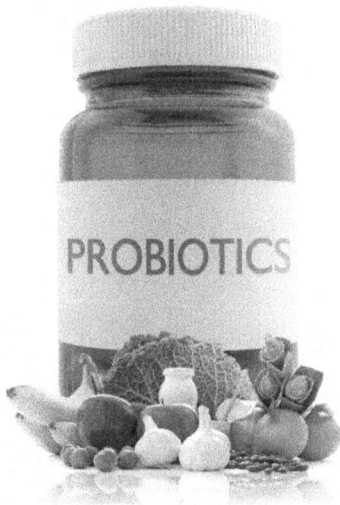

If it is necessary for you to take an antibiotic, we recommend taking all of it as directed and taking a quality multi-strain probiotic for several weeks (or months!) afterward to restore and rebuild a healthy gut flora. We also recommend copious and frequent consumption of fermented foods (pickles, sauerkraut, yogurt, fermented vegetables, Kombucha) for the beneficial bacteria they provide.

AN OUNCE OF PREVENTION ...

It is much easier to prevent contamination or colonization from becoming an infection than to halt one already in progress. Nature provides a cornucopia of botanicals to help resist infection. Natural compounds which can be used topically or systemically that boost your immune system function and help rid you of an infection include oil of oregano, olive leaf extract, garlic, calendula, and Manuka honey. Echinacea, sunlight, and accompanying optimal vitamin D levels (you may want to supplement with it also) are also very important to help optimize your health (as are the measures mentioned previously). Best of all, bacteria do not tend to develop resistance to these natural treatments.

"Here's good advice for practice: go into partnership with nature; she does more than half the work and asks none of the fee."

—Dr. Martin H. Fisher

Recent research has shown that Komodo dragon blood contains an important compound which could be developed into an antibiotic in the future. The compound (DRGN-1) promoted the healing of infected wounds in mice. Far-fetched as this sounds, scientists are continuously on a quest to find new antibiotics to fight multidrug-resistant pathogens.

Even the best antibiotics do not rid you of infections alone. They typically rely on significantly weakening and decreasing the bacterial numbers while your immune system does the rest. Having high blood sugar makes your immune cells sluggish and hampers their ability to fight infection. If you have diabetes, ask your doctor to help you keep your blood sugars tightly controlled as an all-around preventive measure.

The key to keeping your immune system healthy is making good lifestyle choices such as adequate sunlight, proper diet, stress management, lots of sleep, respecting your chronobiology, and exercise. Always opt for clean, whole foods (animal and plant based), organically raised without antibiotics and preferably locally sourced. By taking control of your own health and building a strong immune system, you will minimize your risk of acquiring an antibiotic-resistant infection.

References and Recommended Reading

1. DaCosta RS, Kulbatski I, Lindvere-Teene L, Starr D, Blackmore K, Silver JI, et al. (2015) *Point-of-Care* Autofluorescence Imaging for Real-Time Sampling and Treatment Guidance of Bioburden in Chronic Wounds: *First-in-Human Results*. PLoS ONE 10(3): e0116623. https://doi.org/10.1371/journal.pone.0116623

2. Weng QY, Raff AB, Cohen JM, et al. "Costs and consequences associated with misdiagnosed lower extremity cellulitis." *JAMA Dermatol.* 2016. doi: 10.1001/jamadermatol.2016.3816. [Epub ahead of print]

3. Atttinger C, Wolcott R. "Clinically Addressing Biofilm in Chronic Wounds." *Adv Wound Care (New Rochelle)*. 2012 Jun; 1(3): 127–132.

4. Gardner SE, Frantz RA, Doebbeling BN. "The Validity of the Clinical Signs and Symptoms used to Identify Localized Chronic Wound Infection." *Wound Repair Regen.* 2001 May-Jun;9(3):178-86.

5. Mercola, Joseph. "Bitter Pill: Serious Side Effects of Fluoroquinolone Antibiotics." *Mercola.com.* Dr. Mercola, 1 Nov. 2014. Web. 11 June 2017.

6. "Is Komodo dragon blood the key to new antibiotics?" BBC News. April 12, 2017.

CHAPTER 17

Oxygen Heals

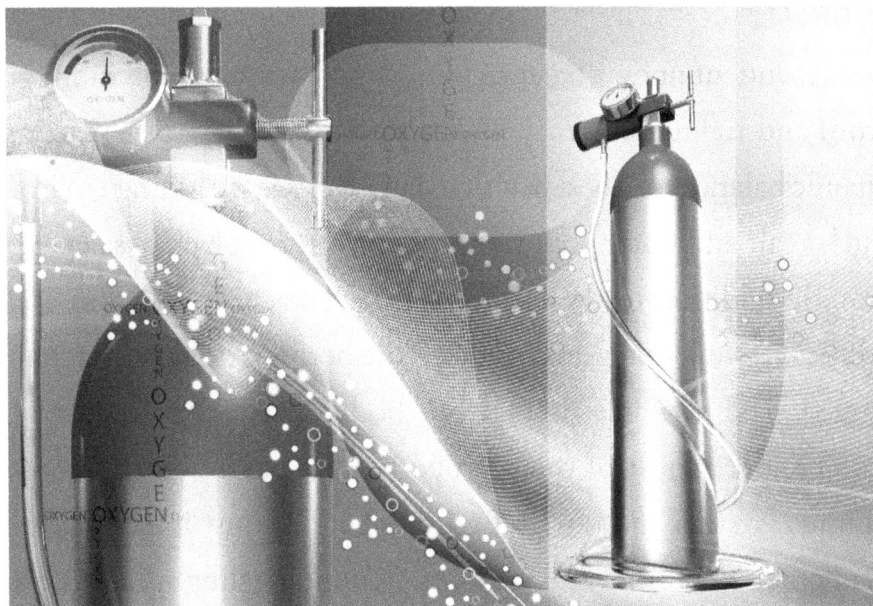

At times, wounds may require surgery or prescription medications. These modalities have their place, and surgeons and pharmaceutical products do excellent work every single day all over the world. Sometimes, however, there are easier, gentler therapies that are non-invasive and have no negative side effects. Some may even work better than conventional treatment or be best applied together with conventional medicine.

Nearly one-third of patients in hospital-based outpatient wound centers may not heal their wounds even though they are cared for over a long period of time. As we have gained more experience with the high costs, inconvenience to the patient, side effects, and often-ineffective medical procedures used to treat chronic wounds, we have become more interested in natural therapies. No better prescription exists than oxygen. Providing more oxygen molecules is one way we discuss here. You have probably heard by now of oxygenated water and oxygen spas. A far more effective way is hyperbaric oxygen. Another less expensive and easier method is to induce oxidation.

BIO-OXIDATIVE THERAPIES

Healing is dependent upon a balance in the body between oxidation (giving up an electron) and reduction (receiving an electron). These two reactions must be in dynamic balance for good health. Many factors, including environmental toxins (such as air and water pollution), poor nutrition, lack of sleep, poor ATP production, in addition to the lack of sunlight reaching our skin and retina, make it difficult to maintain this balance. The body's oxidative systems become overwhelmed. The net effect is that our bodies gradually lose the ability to oxidize toxins and dispose of them properly. This has a negative consequence to the immune system and our ability to defend against infections, allergens, toxins, and other environmental stressors. Wound healing is likewise affected.

Oxidizers like hydrogen peroxide and ozone can stimulate the body's oxidative enzyme systems and return balance, sometimes allowing wounds to heal. Hydrogen peroxide and ozone can be combined in a therapeutic approach known as bio-oxidative therapy.

> "The almost complete lack of adverse side effects places hydrogen peroxide and ozone therapies into a superior class of therapeutic agents never before identified."
>
> —Charles Farr, MD, PhD, Nobel Prize nominee 1993

Bio-oxidative therapies are an integral part of a holistic approach to health. They facilitate the oxidation of viruses and bacteria in addition to weak and sick cells, allowing stronger and healthier cells to take their place. Bio-oxidative therapies accelerate metabolism and stimulate the release of oxygen atoms from the bloodstream to the cells. When tissue oxygen levels increase, the risk of disease and infection decreases. Healthy cells survive and are better able to multiply. Better wound healing is the result.

An international team of researchers in Barcelona recognized that when bacteria form biofilms, they produce toxins that make cells dormant—and antibiotics cannot target dormant cells, and thus antibiotic resistance increases. The researchers found that 10 percent oxygen is sufficient to wake up bacteria, but in a biofilm, only the bacteria on the edges of the film can be reached by oxygen therapy. Those farther inside the film might not get exposed to the oxygen, which would otherwise break up the biofilm and disperse the bacteria. You already know that debridement is necessary to break up biofilm. What if oxygen could be used to help both inhibit the formation of biofilms and, if already present in a wound, break it apart?

1. Hydrogen Peroxide (H_2O_2)

Hydrogen peroxide (H_2O_2) has long been used topically as a disinfectant, antiseptic, and oxidizer. It has a remarkable cleaning and healing effect on the skin. It is manufactured by the body and is involved in all of life's vital processes. It must be present for the immune system to function properly. The cells that fight infection, granulocytes, produce hydrogen peroxide as a first line of defense against invading parasites, viruses, bacteria, and yeast.

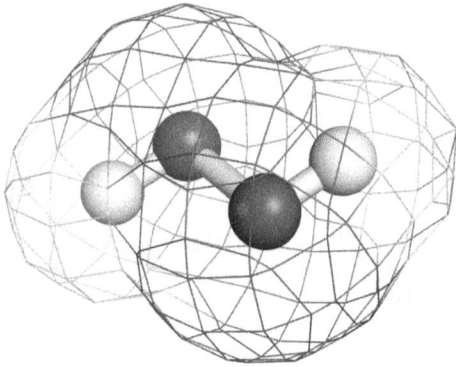

It has many other functions as well, such as helping to metabolize food (breaking down proteins, fats, and carbohydrates to be used as energy) and regulating hormones (such as estrogen, progesterone, and thyroxine). It plays a vital role in regulating blood sugar and the production of energy in all body cells. This link between insulin, metabolized sugar, oxygenation, and hydrogen peroxide produced by your body may be one reason why individuals who have insulin-resistant diabetes heal more slowly.

Most clinicians today do not recommend using antiseptic solutions to clean a chronic wound for the same reason hydrogen peroxide is not recommended. The antiseptic will often destroy your healthy cells, dry out the wound, slow healing, and increase your risk of scar tissue formation. However, if you do need a powerful and effective antiseptic, diluted hydrogen peroxide is our first choice as it is far safer than rubbing (isopropyl) alcohol or Betadine. We do not recommend ingesting (swallowing) hydrogen peroxide, although it can be done safely with appropriate medical supervision and consultation. In high concentrations, this can lead to critical illness and death.

There are some newly recognized non-topical indications for hydrogen peroxide. A study at the Baylor University Medical Center reported in the *American Journal of Surgery* that wounds caused by radiation treatment for cancer healed better after intra-arterial hydrogen peroxide. The researchers attributed this to super-oxygenating the irradiated area via hydrogen peroxide molecules.

Intravenous infusion of hydrogen peroxide has been shown to have a positive metabolic effect. Wounds are often infected with a variety of resistant organisms. Intravenous hydrogen peroxide can help eradicate these infections without the downsides and side effects of intensive antibiotic therapy. It is extremely effective at ridding the body of a variety of pathogenic organisms such as candidiasis (yeast), many bacterial infections, viral infections including influenza and the "common cold," sinus infections, Epstein-Barr virus (EBV), and gangrene.

Intravenous H_2O_2 also helps dissolve vascular plaques. This can help, if given with ethylenediaminetetraacetic acid (EDTA), a commonly used chelating agent, to improve vascular circulation—a key problem with many wounds. The combination of intravenous hydrogen peroxide and EDTA is known as "Chelox Therapy."

2. Ozone (O$_3$)

Ozone (O_3) is an energized and highly reactive form of oxygen with extra electrons. It was first used to disinfect wounds during World War I. It kills bacteria by rupturing their cell walls. Once it enters the body, ozone is reduced to hydrogen peroxide, which produces similar effects.

Ozone is very inexpensive to produce; yet, it is very potent. Drug companies do not want to see it get developed since it would be very difficult for them to compete. We like therapies that can empower our patients and that they can do at home. Inexpensive medical grade ozone generators are

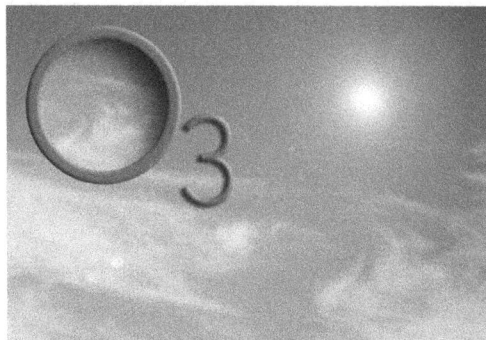

available, and this therapy can easily be applied to non-healing wounds by (plastic) bagging the wounded area and running ozone into the bag.

Ozonated oils have been used in wound care for over a century, and this is a popular and effective therapy in Europe. Ozone gas is added to olive oil and applied as a salve. This helps treat a wide variety of skin problems, including dermatitis, cellulitis, fungal infections, leg ulcers, pressure ulcers, herpes simplex, hemorrhoids, insect bites, acne, hidradenitis suppurativa, and yeast infections (candidiasis). In 1988, scientists at the Pasteur Polyclinic in Havana studied ozonated oil for varicose ulcers. All sixty patients using the ozonated oil were completely healed within fifteen to thirty days, while the control group needed an average of fifty-three days to heal, and a few still had not healed at the end of 155 days. This oil can be easily obtained from a variety of sources and used at home.

Both of these bio-oxidative therapies are safe, effective, natural, and inexpensive adjuncts to help heal wounds. They naturally enhance the immune systems and promote healing.

3. Hyperbaric Oxygen Therapy (HBOT)

This highly effective oxygen therapy might be covered by your insurance company for some specific wound types. HBOT is a method of administering pure oxygen at greater than atmospheric pressure to a patient, which forces the oxygen into the tissues. Although the extra oxygen can help people with numerous conditions, in conventional medicine, it is most widely used to help

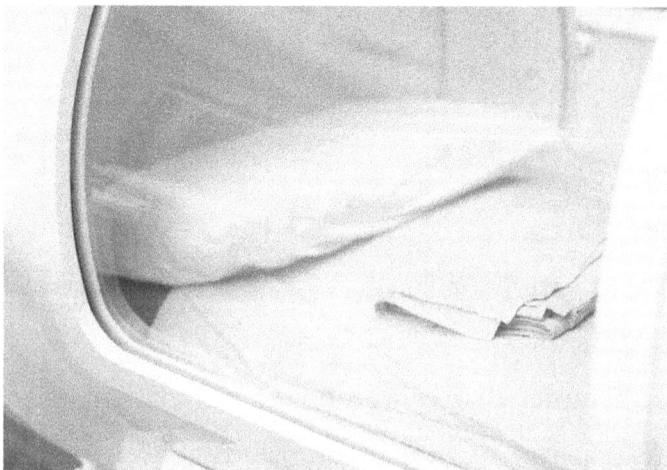

heal difficult wounds. HBOT is very effective when combined with standard wound care. HBOT is a primary treatment for scuba diving accidents, gas gangrene (along with surgery), carbon monoxide poisoning, and radiation injury resulting from cancer treatment (soft tissue radionecrosis and osteoradionecrosis).

HBOT is the best way to deliver oxygen to under-oxygenated tissue and encourages the growth of new tissue. Granulation tissue (the pink, fleshy tissue that first grows over a healing wound) can often be seen within seven to ten days of starting a patient on HBOT. By thirty days, this tissue becomes densely supplied with new blood vessels. Oxygen also promotes the growth of collagen, the material from which skin and connective tissue are formed.

HBOT helps speed the healing of chronic ulcers related to ischemia or diabetes. HBOT increases the oxygen concentration of the blood plasma and lymph, which normally do not carry oxygen. This dissolved oxygen is more readily available to the body than the oxygen which is normally carried by the hemoglobin molecules in the red blood cells. Thus, it promotes the healing of skin ulcers caused by reduced blood flow (PAD). Relief from hypoxia can help relieve the pain experienced by PAD patients. HBOT also reduces the swelling that accompanies hypoxia, making it easier for the affected tissues to rid themselves of toxic cellular wastes.

In addition, HBOT can reduce the incidence and extent of gangrene. This can save an affected limb from amputation. Where amputation is unavoidable, the use of HBOT can help delineate which tissue is healthy and which is dead, thus allowing the surgeon to save as much viable tissue and as much of the limb as possible.

HBOT helps minimize tissue death, decrease swelling, and reduce the chance of infection. It also encourages bone repair in cases of osteomyelitis (bone infection). The cells that repair bone depend on a rich supply of oxygen.

HBOT also helps kill anaerobic bacteria and helps antibiotics such as sulfa drugs work more effectively.

Finally, HBOT helps reverse the damage caused by radiation therapy, which causes severe tissue hypoxia. The location of the damage depends on where the cancer under treatment was located. Radiation damages both the skin and soft tissues (soft-tissue radionecrosis) and sometimes the bone (osteo-radionecrosis). The late effects of radiation can also cause problems with the bladder, prostate gland, and rectum (radiation cystitis, prostatitis, and proctitis, respectively). Hyperbaric oxygen has been documented to be one of the only helpful therapies for these truly miserable conditions. Radiation proctitis has also been reported to be responsive to local ozone therapy.

If you have any of these medical conditions, you should find the nearest hyperbaric medicine center and schedule a consultation.

HBOT is the mainstay of therapy in most hospital-affiliated and insurance-billing wound centers. Unfortunately, most wound centers are constrained by the necessity of insurance reimbursement and will not be able to offer HBOT to patients whose wounds would benefit unless they meet very specific criteria. In our experience, HBOT would be incredibly helpful to a much larger number of patients than those who qualify to have their insurance reimburse it.

HBOT can be administered to patients in either monoplace or multi-place chambers—monoplace meaning only one person at a time can be in the chamber, and multiplace meaning the chamber can fit several people. Usually there is an attendant who "dives" with the patient in multiplace chambers, and many people prefer multiplace chambers because they get less claustro-phobic. The newer monoplace chambers are actually quite roomy and are mostly window space to minimize the feeling of claustrophobia. Safety is also an important consideration since pure oxygen is very combustible, and there are several important rules that must be followed to safely use a hyperbaric chamber.

There are home hyperbaric chambers available also, but be aware of the limitations—you cannot pressurize them anywhere near as much as a commercial grade chamber; therefore, therapy will not be as effective. Nonetheless, they can be either purchased or leased from a variety of sources and may be the best alternative for you if you do not have access to a real, commercial grade chamber or if your insurance will not allow commercial grade HBOT. Again, you need to pay close attention to safety issues and make sure you read and follow all of the precautions/documentation that accompany the product you end up using.

Many doctors do not know about HBOT because they do not learn about it in medical school. Despite a massive volume of scientific data on the subject, the field is still young. Since hyperbaric chambers use only oxygen as their therapy and are quite expensive to manufacture, acquire, maintain, and operate, there is little money to be made by researching further uses of hyperbaric oxygen as opposed to all the potential profits to be made by mass-manufacturing new pharmaceuticals.

Many hyperbaric doctors believe that HBOT can be used for many more conditions, including acute or chronic head injuries, migraines, near drowning, strokes, heart attacks, Lyme disease, autism, cerebral palsy, spinal cord injury, various sports injuries, and multiple sclerosis. In addition, some plastic surgeons have found that their patients recover more quickly after surgery with the use of HBOT. These additional applications have yet to be FDA-approved or accepted by insurance companies, but there are many small studies documenting efficacy in all these applications. Unlike pharmaceuticals where a real medication can be given to one group and a placebo to another group, it is difficult to "placebo-control" a study of HBOT.

We believe that as more doctors learn about the benefits of HBOT, more of them will recommend this highly effective treatment. HBOT is safe and non-invasive and could produce savings on other therapies that would be in the millions and maybe billions of dollars and vastly improve the lives of many who have conditions that are not currently particularly responsive to other treatments. We hope that this book will stimulate readers to discuss hyperbaric medicine with their friends, doctors, and local hospitals, so that more HBOT centers will become available, more diagnoses will be covered, and more patients will benefit from the healing effects of hyperbaric oxygen. Some entrepreneurial physicians, naturopaths, and chiropractors have started their own "cash-based" hyperbaric treatment centers that offer the therapy at more reasonable prices than the typical insurance-billing wound center.

One hyperbaric nurse says, "HBOT is a slow process, but I see how much it changes patient lives. Numerous patients said they thought they had to live with their difficult symptoms and pain. Some were told there was nothing more that could be done for them. When these patients begin to see progress, I am overwhelmingly grateful. It is almost as if each healed wound ignites an epiphany—our patients have hope again." [Holmes, Chimere. Inside HBOT: A Nurse's Story, *Ostomy Wound Management*, March 2011; 57 (3); 18-19.]

References and Recommended Reading

1. Lane, Nick. *Oxygen: The Molecule That Made the World.* Oxford, United Kingdom: Oxford UP, 2016. Print.

2. Neubauer, Richard E., and Morton Walker. *Hyperbaric Oxygen Therapy: Using HBO Therapy to Increase Circulation, Repair Damaged Tissue, Fight Infection, Save Limbs, Relieve Pain, and More.* Garden City Park, NY: Avery, 1998. Print.

3. Altman, Nathaniel. *Oxygen Healing Therapies: For Optimum Health & Vitality: Bio-oxidative Therapies for Treating Immune Disorders, Candida, Cancer, Heart, Skin, Circulatory & Other Modern Diseases.* Rochester, VT: Healing Arts, 1998. Print.

4. Fife CE. "Is HBOT cost-effective for diabetic foot ulcers?" *Podiatry Today.* 2009; 22(6).

5. Messer, A'ndrea Elyse. "Oxygen Can Wake up Dormant Bacteria for Antibiotic Attacks." *Penn State University.* Penn State News, 8 Dec. 2016. Web. 11 June 2017.

6. Thom SR, Bhopale VM, Velazquez OC, Goldstein LJ, Thom LH, Buerk DG (April 2006). "Stem cell mobilization by hyperbaric oxygen". American Journal of Physiology. Heart and Circulatory Physiology. 290 (4): H1378–H1386. PMID 16299259. doi:10.1152/ajpheart.00888.2005.

CHAPTER 18

Advanced and Alternative Therapies

The longer we practice alternative therapies, the more aware we become of a variety of issues that prevent the body from healing. Chronic wounds often need advanced and alternative therapies to wake up dysfunctional cells or supply additional energy to the body to help it heal. This might be the only way to finally achieve tissue repair and regeneration.

We want to share with you some advanced and alternative methods (besides oxygen) that can make all the difference in healing your chronic wound. Although these methods are not really *secrets*, they are often ignored or unknown by mainstream medicine. You will not find them at a conventional wound center since they are not reimbursed by insurance. We combine these advanced therapies for especially hard to heal wounds. Customizing individual treatment programs is the *art* of wound care medicine.

1. DETOXIFICATION

Today more than ever, we live in an environment with a number of toxic challenges to our biology. Collectively, these conditions can prevent wounds from healing and have an adverse impact on overall health. We have previously discussed the importance of drinking a lot of good quality (non-fluoridated reverse osmosis filtered or spring) water. Drinking water not only helps build exclusion zones in your cells but also helps your body flush out toxins through the kidneys, sweating, tears, and bowel movements. The worse your diet (think genetically modified organisms [GMOs]), the more toxins you need to get rid of.

We have found that many of our patients have heavy metal toxicities. Lead can displace the trace mineral zinc in tissues, which can lead to impaired healing (recall the importance of zinc for healing). Lead is also known to be a significant neurotoxin and can lead to many adverse effects on your brain. Other potential sources of metal toxicity are silver amalgam dental fillings (mercury), vaccines and cookware (aluminum), and paint and pottery glaze (lead). Eating conventionally raised (as opposed to organic) meat introduces artificial hormones, antibiotics, pesticides, and herbicides. Conventionally raised (non-organic) fruits and vegetables may contain herbicides and pesticides. Contaminated water supplies may have halogens (like chlorine, fluorine, and bromine), industrial waste, runoff from crops and fields (pesticides and herbicides along with fertilizer), and waste pharmaceuticals.

Toxins also come from a host of environmental sources including everyday cleaning products. For some, careers such as printing, manufacturing, art, and chemistry may put them in regular contact with toxic chemicals and heavy metals. Environmental air pollutants, particularly in populous areas, can be a very significant health hazard. Every breath can be an exposure to a variety of toxins, which can eventually accumulate and have a significant biologic effect.

A urine challenge test can be used to determine the presence of most heavy metals. If present, then chelation therapy, usually with a combination of intra-venous and oral agents, can be life-changing. Heavy metals are chelated from the blood vessels and tissues and excreted. Some patients concur-rently receive a "Meyer's cocktail" (a fortified intravenous vitamin mixture) to restore essential minerals lost during chelation. Chelation can be very helpful in peripheral arterial disease, which significantly impairs healing. This can obviate the need for surgery, stents, or drugs. "Increased flow to the toes, the leg doesn't go."

2. LIGHT THERAPY

As has been pointed out in Chapter 8, light is essential to life, and light can have a tremendous effect on biology.

Low-level light therapy (LLLT) is the application of light to the body to promote tissue regeneration, reduce inflammation, and relieve pain. Typically, a laser (monochromatic light) in the red and or near-infrared spectrum is used. LLLT exerts a photochemical effect, like photosynthesis in plants, whereby the light is absorbed and exerts a chemical change. This is a type of photobiomodulation, which means using photons to modulate biological activity. LLLT has been used for many years on sports injuries, arthritic joints, and back and neck pain. Studies have now shown that light is effective in the treatment of open wounds when it is used as a component of a total wound management program.

In addition to "traditional" LLLT which typically uses monochromatic (single frequency) light, there is now tremendous promise shown by a device being developed by a company called PhotoMed Technologies that sweeps through a range of specific frequencies. In fact, preliminary work has demonstrated that some wounds exposed to a device of this type can literally be observed to undergo angiogenesis (new blood vessel formation) and form granulation tissue while being exposed to the treatment in the clinic. Although this device is still in the experimental stage, we hope it will soon be available for general use and will be keeping a close eye on it.

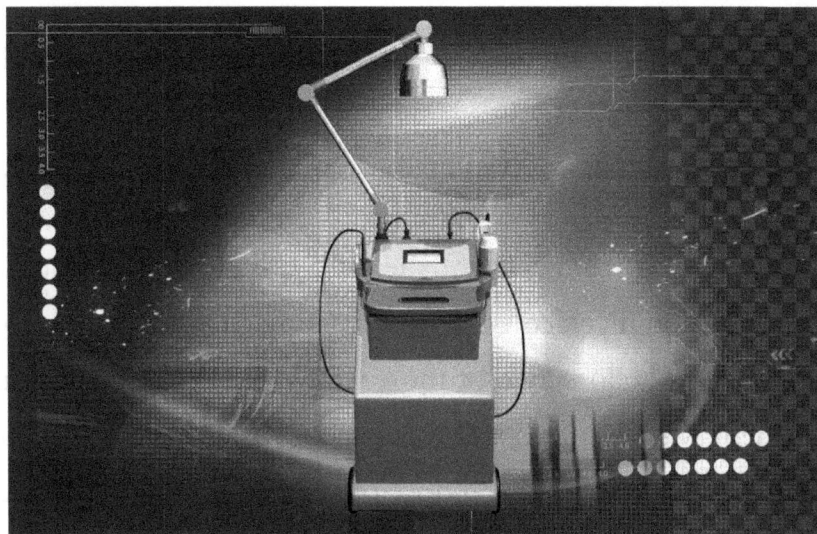

How does it work?

As we have discussed, cells are extremely responsive to light, and certain frequencies/wavelengths can very much influence how proteins in the mitochondrial respiratory transport chain (responsible for the bodies energy production) work. Those wavelengths, when applied to a wound, can increase adenosine triphosphate (ATP) production and have been found to promote rapid granulation and wound repair. The photons, which are produced by lasers or light-emitting diodes, are absorbed by the cells of injured skin (these cells are more sensitive than those of intact tissue). Once absorbed, a cascade of biochemical events occurs. The mitochondria, essentially the power plants of the cell, may produce more ATP, helping tissues heal more quickly. LLLT improves tissue repair and reduces inflammation and pain wherever the beam is directed. The ultimate result is accelerated wound healing and healing of ulcers that fail to respond to other forms of treatment.

"The use of low levels of visible or near infrared light for reducing pain, inflammation and edema, promoting healing of wounds, deeper tissues and nerves, and preventing cell death and tissue damage has been known for over forty years."

—Professor Michael Hamblin, Harvard-MIT Division of Health Sciences and Technology

---

If you are suffering from a venous leg ulcer, diabetic foot ulcer, pressure ulcer, or post-radiation ulcer, consider this therapy. Treatments take only a few minutes and are usually done two or more times a week. Debridement should precede treatment with LLLT to stimulate acute inflammation and expose the viable tissue to the highest potential dose of the incident light. This combination stimulates granulation to form and helps with wound contracture.

One such LLLT device, the THOR laser, has been extensively studied and is very effective. Another device, the Delta Laser, has multiple frequencies and includes magnetic and ultrasound therapy. It has been shown to be remarkably helpful at speeding wound healing and helping wounds which otherwise would not heal get significant traction towards closure.

Acute and chronic radiation-induced dermatitis can occur after high doses of radiation for cancer treatment. Sometimes the dermatitis progresses to soft tissue radionecrosis with ulcer formation. Chronic radiation ulcers are one of the hardest to heal wound types. There are case reports of patients with long-lasting radiation ulcers which finally healed thanks to LLLT. A video measuring the number of dermal vessels in the ulcer before and after LLLT showed a statistically significant increase in the number of dermal vessels, both in the central and marginal parts of the wound, compared with its pretreatment status. The more blood vessels present, the better the blood flow, the more likely a wound is to heal.

Using LLLT *in conjunction with* PRP and stem cell therapy can produce very impressive results.

There is a therapeutic window in the range of red and near infrared light where the efficiency of light penetration in the tissue is maximal. This phototherapy can stimulate stem cells and promote healing of wounds. LLLT devices are simple to use and very cost-effective. More importantly, they improve the quality of life for patients. There is a variety of other conditions that they can significantly improve, including chronic pain and depression, both distressingly common in patients with non-healing wounds.

A somewhat less expensive variant of this that you can try at home is to procure a panel of red LEDs in the 650–680nm (nanometer) wavelength range and shine that on your wounds. Several companies make arrays of LEDs in this range, and there is a variety of other sources. The 650nm wavelength is known to be a very healing frequency and directly stimulates the cytochromes in the respiratory transport chain of mitochondria. Another frequency known to stimulate healing is 380 nm in the ultraviolet range. You must be more careful with this, as it carries a lot more energy than the red light and could potentially cause burns or other harm with overexposure.

Combining red light therapy with methylene blue dressings provides even more potent bactericidal effects. Studies have shown that methylene blue plus potassium iodide combined with red light is even more bactericidal and prevents recurrent infection. This suggests that light can be an "antibiotic" to which bacteria cannot become resistant. Given the problem of drug-resistant infections, this is excellent news.

3. MICROCURRENT

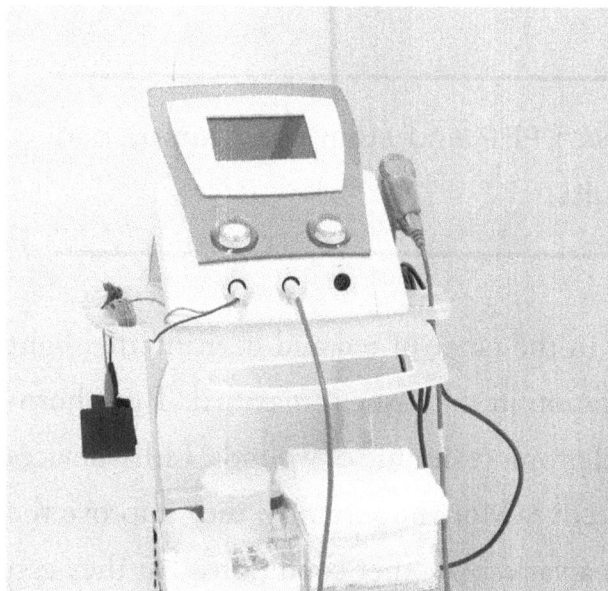

Simply put, our bodies are electric. You are certainly aware that every beat of your heart is initiated and controlled by a precisely timed electrical current—doctors measure this when they do an ECG—electrocardiogram. Likewise, thoughts formed in your brain are carried by electric currents, and electric signals travel down nerves to control your muscles. There is nothing in your body that does not somehow depend on electricity. As we have previously discussed, this should certainly give you pause to consider just how "safe" manmade electromagnetic fields (EMF) are for your health.

Doctors have known for many years that electricity can be used in a therapeutic manner to help heal the body. For example, specific electric currents have been used to accelerate bone healing in fractures that are not healing (orthopedists refer to this as "non-union"). TENS therapy (transcutaneous electrical nerve stimulation) has been used for many years to control both acute and chronic pain.

Many tissues in your body are conductors or semi-conductors; for example, bone is a semi-conductor. Much of this was proven and some important work on this was done by Dr. Robert Becker, an orthopedic surgeon who studied such diverse topics as salamander limb regeneration and bone healing. He was truly a pioneer in helping us to understand that the human body operates by way of electric currents, something that is largely in the blind spot of mainstream medicine.

Enter microcurrent. Frequency specific microcurrent electrical therapy (FSM, also known as MET [microcurrent electrical therapy]) uses current

1,000 times less than that of TENS, but the pulse is 2,500 times longer than the pulse in a typical TENS unit. This improves pain control and accelerates wound healing. FSM is useful for a variety of problems including many pain-related disorders, providing relief of symptoms and quickly promoting healing. Unlike pharmaceuticals, it has no side effects. Most physicians are unaware of the therapeutic benefit of FSM.

"Use of MET is simple, safe, and efficient and can have tremendous influence on improving wound healing."

—Dr. Joseph Mercola

How does it work?

A small micro-electric, direct current generator at low frequency is applied directly to a wound site through a composite wound dressing. An electric potential difference is established between an anode and cathode of the composite wound dressing. Wound healing is enhanced by the biostimulatory effect of the applied microcurrent, which increases ATP production, cell membrane transport of amino acids, and protein synthesis.

Additional studies have found that direct electrical therapy stimulates fibroblasts to secrete growth factor, a major regulator of cell-mediated inflammation and tissue regeneration. Substances that increase electrical field, such as prostaglandin E2, enhance the wound healing rate and increase cell division. Electrical fields stimulate secretion of growth factor. Low frequency current stimulates ATP production. Sound familiar? Another study showed that microcurrent stimulates dermal fibroblasts to secrete transforming growth factor-β, a major regulator of cell-mediated inflammation and tissue regeneration.

Significant acceleration of the healing process after microcurrent electrical stimulation has been widely documented. After sustaining a skin and tissue injury, the cell membrane electric potential is altered in the injured tissue. A current of injury occurs, and this triggers repair. The "injury signal" gradually decreases in parallel to the repair process and ceases when the repair is complete. The voltage peaks immediately after injury and gradually decreases as the wound heals. Therefore, the theory is that current flow may be defective in chronic wounds and that applying electrical currents to wounds may stimulate healing.

Electrical stimulation via electrodes placed on the skin adjacent to or directly within the wound, has become an advanced wound care modality. The epidermis maintains a "skin battery" that generates an endogenous electric field and current flow when wounded. Experimental models have demonstrated that most of the cell types within the wound can sense an electric field and respond with a variety of biological and functional responses that can contribute to healing.

Electrical stimulation of a wound increases the concentration of growth factor receptors which increases collagen formation. "This is the first demonstration, in diabetic wounds or any chronic wounds, that the naturally occurring electrical signal is impaired and correlated with delayed wound healing. Correcting this defect offers a totally new approach for chronic and non-healing wounds in diabetes.

In late 2015, a team from Washington State University found that antibiotics could be replaced by electrical stimulation, and that this new method was often more effective. Several months earlier, a team from the UK discovered that healing rates could be sped up via electrical currents. In fact, it took just two weeks of treatment to heal wounds entirely.

Having healed wounds with the help of microcurrent, suffice it to say that it improves healing by facilitating the reestablishment of the subtle electric currents that become disrupted when a wound occurs.

4. BEMER (*B*io - *E*lectro - *M*agnetic - *E*nergy – *R*egulation)

BEMER therapy causes an interaction between the body's cells and a weak pulsating electromagnetic field (of about the same order of magnitude as that of the earth's magnetic field). The effect of this pulsed electromagnetic field on the body takes place at a cellular level. The human body is an agglomeration of basic building blocks, which we call cells, which are self-regulating and self-healing. BEMER activates each cell's biochemical processes and improves energy levels of the cells. It enhances the body's own healing mechanisms.

What are the benefits?

- *Improves micro- and macro-circulation*

- *Improves oxygenation of the blood*

- *Improves elasticity of the blood vessels*

- *Improves wound healing and regeneration*

- *Strengthens the immune system*

Blood is essential for life. Without adequate microcirculation, we cannot facilitate the exchange of nutrients and waste products between the blood and tissues. Without blood comes oxygen deprivation, a shortage of ATP, and minimal cellular energy. Not to mention pain! As a wound management specialist working in an advanced wound management center, I can tell you that most chronic wounds, whether from venous insufficiency, arterial insufficiency, lymphedema, diabetes, auto-immune disease, or non-healing surgical wounds, etc., have an underlying circulatory disorder at their core. Improved vascular flow cannot be underestimated in wound healing, and not all patients can or want to undergo a vascular procedure or bypass surgery.

The BEMER device has the unique ability to enhance delivery of nutrients and oxygen while removing waste material from the blood. The BEMER technology has enabled us to provide the best possible care for the compromised patients that we treat. Diabetic patients with neuropathy often experience improvement in sensation. This technology is invaluable in patients with microvascular disorders or insufficiency and has been shown to assist in saving limbs. There are no contra-indications or negative side effects from BEMER treatment.

Many papers about electromagnetic field therapy have been published in international medical journals in the past fifteen years. These describe their remarkably high degree of efficacy in wound and fracture healing.

References and Recommended Reading

1. Tuner, Jan. *Laser Therapy: Clinical Practice and Scientific Background; a Guide for Research Scientists, Doctors, Dentists, Veterinarians and Other Interested Parties within the Medical Field.* GrÃ¤ngesberg: Prima, 2002. Print. 189–96.

2. Isseroff, R. Rivkah, and Sara E. Dahle. "Electrical Stimulation Therapy and Wound Healing: Where Are We Now?" *Advances in Wound Care* 1.6 (2012): 238–243. *PMC.* Web. 11 June 2017.

3. Mester, E., Mester, A. F. and Mester, A. (1985), "The biomedical effects of laser application." *Lasers Surg. Med.,* 5: 31–39. doi:10.1002/lsm.1900050105: 31-9.

4. Barbor, Meg. "Low-Level Laser Therapy Ameliorates Radiation Dermatitis." *Medscape.* Medscape, 16 July 2015. Web. 11 June 2017.

5. Wilson, Clare. "Burst of Light Speeds up Healing by Turbocharging Our Cells." *New Scientist.* 10 July 2015. Web. 11 June 2017.

6. "Low-level light stirs in vivo stem cells to regenerate tissue." *BioOptics World.* 29 July 2014. Web 11 June 2017.

7. Morison, Moya. *The Prevention and Treatment of Pressure Ulcers*. New York: Mosby, 2001. 177–93. Print.

8. https://www.thorlaser.com/wound/Mary-Dyson.pdf. Web.

9. http://www.lasertherapeutics.us/papers/Mary%20Dyson%20Laser%20Therapy.pdf. Web.

10. http://photobiology.info/Hamblin.html. Web.

11. S. Young, P. Bolton, M. Dyson, W. Harvey and C. Diamantopoulos, "Macrophage responsiveness to light therapy." Lasers Surg Med 9 (1989) 497–505.

12. Hopkins, J. Ty et al. "Low-Level Laser Therapy Facilitates Superficial Wound Healing in Humans: A Triple-Blind, Sham-Controlled Study." *Journal of Athletic Training* 39.3 (2004): 223–229. Print.

13. Kloth LC. "Electrical stimulation for wound healing: a review of evidence from in vitro studies, animal experiment, and clinical trials." *Int J Low Extrem Wounds.* 2005; 4(1): 23–44.

14. McGinnis ME, Vanable JW. "Voltage gradients in newt limb stumps." *Prog Clin Biol Res.* 1986; 210: 231-8.

15. Becker, Robert O., and Gary Selden. *The Body Electric*. New York: Morrow, 1998. Print.

16. Basset CA. "Beneficial effects of electromagnetic fields." *J Cell Biochem.* 1993; 51(4): 387–93.

17. Cheng N, et al. "The effects of electric currents on ATP generation, protein synthesis, and membrane transport of rat skin." *Clin Orthop Relat Res.* 1982; 171: 264-72.

18. Zhao M, et al. "Electrical stimulation directly induces pre-angiogenic response in vascular endothelial cells by signaling through VEGF receptors." *J Cell Sci.* 2003; 117: 397–405

19. Todd I, et al. "Electrical stimulation of transforming growth factor-beta 1 secretion by human dermal fibroblasts and the U937 human monocytic cell line." *Altern Lab Anim.* 2001; 29: 693–701

20. Mercola JM, Kirsch DL. "The Basis for Microcurrent Electrical Therapy in Conventional Medical Practice." *J Adv in Med.* 1995; 8 (2): 83–152.

21. Schindl A, et al. "Increased dermal angiogenesis after low-intensity laser therapy for a chronic radiation ulcer determined by a video measuring system." *J Am Acad Dermatol* 1999 Mar; 40(3): 481–4.

22. "Electrical Stimulation Could Improve Wound Healing Process." *Advanced Tissue.* N.p., 27 Jan. 2016. Web. 11 June 2017.

23. Naude L. Independent evaluation of BEMER physical vascular regulation therapy. *The Specialist Forum*; June 2013: 9–13.

24. Vecchio, Daniela et al. "Bacterial Photodynamic Inactivation Mediated by Methylene Blue and Red Light Is Enhanced by Synergistic Effect of Potassium Iodide." *Antimicrobial Agents and Chemotherapy* 59.9 (2015): 5203–5212. *PMC.* Web. 11 June 2017.

25. www.PubMed.gov/ Bemer vascular therapy.

26. Verdote-Robertson, Rosario, Michelle M. Munchua, and John R. Reddon. "The Use of Low Intensity Laser Therapy (LILT) for the Treatment of Open Wounds in Psychogeriatric Patients." *Physical & Occupational Therapy In Geriatrics* 18.2 (2000): 1–19. Web.

CHAPTER 19

Regenerative Medicine: Your Body's Own Repair Kit

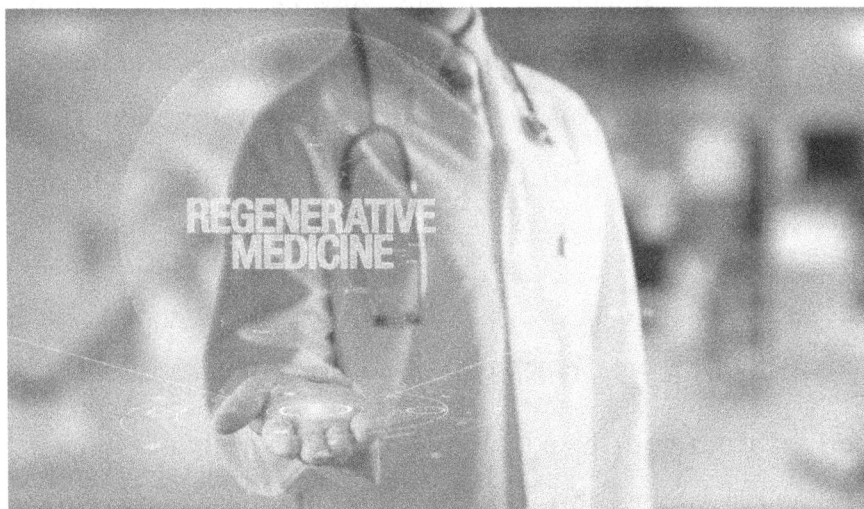

"Think how many people have non-healing chronic wounds, and there is no reason for it! Stem cells will heal those wounds."

—Dr. Sharon McQuillan, Ageless Regenerative Institute

Regenerative medicine is a new field of medicine that is ushering in an era of effective treatment by harnessing the body's own capacity for healing many serious and chronic conditions which have defied traditional medical techniques. Regenerative medicine is defined as "the process of replacing or regenerating human cells, tissues, or organs to restore or establish normal function."

We are on the cusp of many new medical innovations through stem cell therapy. These treatments are helping to repair damaged hearts, restore sight, cure diabetes, and heal burns. Already doctors have used stem cells to grow new vessels that bring blood to dying tissue. They have coaxed stem cells into becoming insulin-secreting beta cells of the pancreas in diabetics. Stem cell therapy is poised to revolutionize wound healing as well.

Two of the most well-known and accessible techniques of the regenerative medicine field are platelet rich plasma therapy (PRP) and stem cell therapy (SCT). We would like to introduce you to the concepts behind these fascinating healing methodologies so you can consider them for helping to heal your wound. If you have been treated by a wound care center, received many advanced modalities already, and your wound remains unhealed, we absolutely recommend these therapies. In our experience, they sometimes work when nothing else will.

PLATELET RICH PLASMA (PRP)

PRP is derived from your own bloodstream so there is no foreign body to react to and no risk of rejection. Your blood is composed of a liquid substance known as plasma (which is mostly water) but also has many important proteins suspended in it and three main types of cells: red blood cells (usually 35-50 percent of the volume of blood), white blood cells (which are an important part of the immune system), and platelets. Most people think of platelets as just important for helping the blood clot in the case of an injury. However, platelets are integral to the important initiating steps in the complex cascade that helps to heal wounds and injuries. They contain many very important growth factors and other cytokines (chemicals secreted by cells), which stimulate healing through a multi-step process.

Cytokines and growth factors included in platelets include the following: platelet derived growth factor, transforming growth factor beta, fibroblast growth factor, insulin-like growth factors 1 and 2, vascular endothelial growth factor, epidermal growth factor, interleukin B, keratinocyte growth factor, and connective tissue growth factor. Just by the names you can recognize that many of these would be very helpful for wound healing, and in fact, these cytokines are crucial to cellular communication and cumulatively accelerate tissue, wound, and bone healing. In addition, they attract and activate stem cells local to the area of injury and encourage them to differentiate and heal the injury.

PRP is simply plasma which has a much higher concentration of platelets than is normally found in the plasma (usually about five to seven times as high, although it can vary depending on the method of production). PRP is easily produced from a patient's own blood using a special centrifuge that spins and separates blood components and isolates the platelets. For the best results, it is important to use a tested and validated protocol and method. It can take as little as twenty minutes to produce PRP and once produced, the

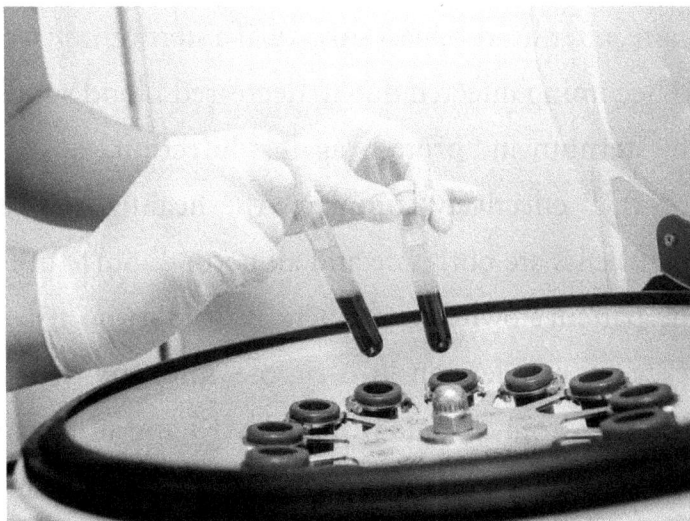

PRP is on top after centrifuging vials of blood

PRP can be activated by specific frequencies of light (no surprise there!) and can be administered back to the injured area, usually by injection into the wound bed and often application to the wound bed as a liquid or gel.

PRP therapy has been found to be very effective for treating a wide variety of common musculoskeletal conditions including acute strains, sprains, muscle tears, partial tendon tears, arthritic joints, and of course chronic wounds. In the case of wounds, PRP can be both injected into and around the area of the wound bed and spread throughout the wound itself.

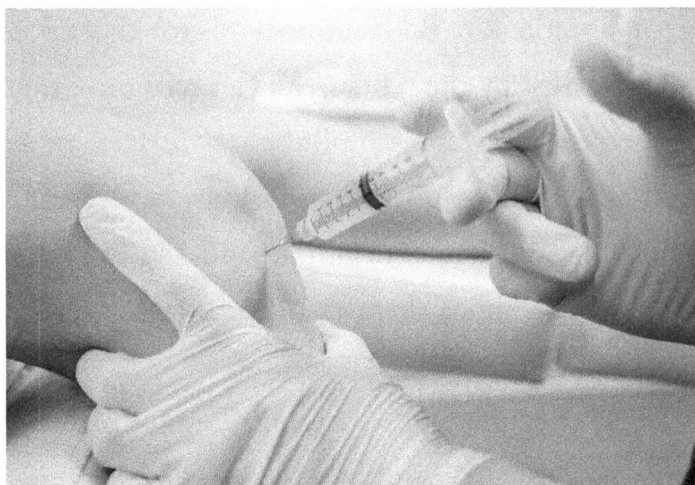

Injecting PRP into a painful knee joint

PRP has helped heal some of the toughest wounds. It can help regrow tissue and skin over exposed bone on feet and ankles. Furthermore, after heart bypass surgery, if a sternotomy wound is healing poorly at risk of becoming infected due to decreased blood supply, PRP promotes healing of the sternum and protects against infection.

PRP effectively stimulates the healing and regeneration of tissues. PRP treatments are both safe and all natural. Since the platelets are harvested from the patient's own blood, there is little to no risk of adverse reaction, allergic reaction, or rejection. It is simple, safe, and delivers lasting benefits for those suffering from chronic wounds. MRI and ultrasound images have proven that PRP therapy results in significant tissue repair in orthopedic conditions, and this tissue repair is obvious to the naked eye in wound healing.

PRP is not like using a drug that goes away after a few half-lives—it activates the body's own potential for healing and creates new blood vessel growth, tissue formation, and changes the character of the wound entirely—and the results accrue over a period of days, weeks, and months. Sometimes multiple applications of PRP are needed to get the best results, but the results can be impressive.

Although PRP has been shown to be extremely effective in wound healing, it is not offered in wound centers because it is not currently reimbursed (in the U.S.) by Medicare or most insurance companies, although it is being considered for reimbursement. Like many effective alternative therapies, this may be because it is difficult (or even impossible) to procure funding for a large, double-blinded, randomized, placebo controlled trial. Although these sorts of trials are easy to do for drugs (that can be very profitable as they can be manufactured in large quantities), the production of PRP is an individualized, time-consuming, and patient specific process (and the efficacy depends on the patient's own baseline platelet counts, which individually vary), and therefore does not lend itself to these sorts of trials which are currently considered the "gold standard" in medicine. For this reason, and despite its proven benefits, most insurance companies still consider it "experimental" and, as you know, they do everything they can to avoid reimbursing things under that category.

It may be possible for you to find a local physician who can prepare PRP and apply it to your wound, and the price will likely vary depending on the market and economics of your area. Many physicians are now starting to use it for cosmetic and orthopedic procedures. We have seen significant benefit from PRP in most stalled and non-healing wounds, but the benefit is best leveraged by careful and expert debridement prior to the application of the PRP—removing the bio-burden and biofilms is crucial to preparing the wound for PRP administration and getting the best results. The combination of expert debridement and PRP use has been shown to be more efficient, cost effective, and convenient for patients than wound vac therapy.

PRP is best used as part of a comprehensive program, and it is a cornerstone of our practice. We have developed a special formulation of PRP—mixed with ozone. In addition, we use specific frequencies of light to "activate" the PRP/ozone mixture, which augments the healing effect *even more*. It is almost magical!

STEM CELL THERAPY (SCT)

You have very likely heard about stem cell therapy and may have heard that it has tremendous potential for wound healing. You may first be wondering what stem cells are and how they can be used therapeutically.

Stem cells (of which there are many types in the body) are precursor cells, which have not yet differentiated, found in many places in the body. They can turn into virtually any necessary cell type, and the type of cell they turn into is controlled by the needs of the local environment in which they find themselves. For example, if a stem cell finds itself in a badly arthritic and inflamed joint lacking cartilage, it is able to reproduce and turn into the necessary cartilage cells to heal the joint and decrease the arthritis pain.

Alternatively, if injected into the bloodstream, stem cells will settle at sites of injury, illness, and inflammation and can become whatever type of cells the body needs to heal itself. They can transform into tissue of various types when the body sends out biochemical signals which activate these cells. They aid in the repair and regrowth of damaged or aging tissues. All of us have trillions of stem cells in our bodies, and they are really what helps us heal and repair our bodies naturally. Stem cell therapy simply seeks to extract those cells, concentrate them, and deliver them back to the place where healing is necessary.

Doctors divide stem cells into two broad categories with respect to their source: autologous (from the patient themselves) and allogeneic (from another person). Both sources have their advantages and disadvantages. Advantages of autologous stem cell therapy include the fact that there is no chance of the body rejecting its own tissue, and there is no risk of contracting an infectious disease (that you don't already have) if the procedure is done carefully. However, some of the advantages of allogeneic stem cells include the fact that your stem cells are as old as you are and sometimes may have been affected by the various toxins and environmental influences that made you ill to start with. That is, an eighty-year-old's stem cells may not be as healthy, vital, and able to reproduce and differentiate as well as cells from a younger person. In addition, sometimes cell number yields during autologous harvesting from older people are lower than hoped for.

In fact, even now there are companies that will "bank" your stem cells, usually by cryogenically preserving them (using a special complex procedure to freeze the cells) so that you can have your own "younger" cells available to you later in life should you need them to combat a disease, injury, or illness. We highly recommend you consider this.

There has been significant controversy regarding stem cell therapy in the public and lay press. This is largely due to the fact some research on stem cells has been done on cells obtained from embryonic sources, typically from discarded or unborn fetuses from terminated pregnancies. A discussion of the religious, moral, and ethical ramifications of using those cell types is well beyond this book, and we do not use these cell types. Rather, the stem cell therapy we focus on and use is autologous therapy, that is, cells obtained from a person's own body, concentrated, and then given back to them.

Stem cell therapy has been around for over fifty years. You have probably heard of patients with certain blood cancers getting bone marrow transplants. Bone marrow transplants are essentially stem cell therapy, using hematopoietic stem cells (cells which produce different types of blood cells), harvested from the bone marrow.

WOUND CENTERS AND SCT

Currently, many wound centers can apply specific engineered tissue products (usually made from amniotic membranes that may contain some stem cells) to wounds and be reimbursed by insurance companies to do so. Although this is not true "stem cell therapy," it is somewhat similar as some of those cells can differentiate into new skin and tissue. Many patients who previously would have required surgical skin grafts have benefitted from these therapies.

Although these therapies can be very effective for many types of wounds, unfortunately, many

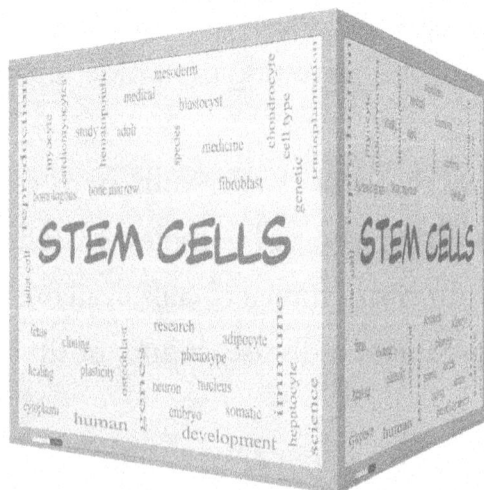

patients do not qualify to have this type of therapy paid for by their insurance for their particular wound. Furthermore, it usually takes multiple applications over weeks or months to heal a wound completely.

PREPARING YOURSELF AND THE WOUND FOR STEM CELL THERAPY

Biochemical signals recruit stem cells to the wound bed and facilitate healing by causing differentiation into the specialized cells required for tissue repair, provided they exist in sufficient numbers and receive the correct signals when injury occurs. When they do not, the result is an inadequate healing response. Stem cell activity can be improved by removing the impediments to new cell creation and proliferation. How? We have outlined all the ways in the preceding chapters (removing high levels of heavy metals, optimizing circadian biology, maximizing light therapy, eating foods that support cell growth and multiplication, hormone optimization, and taking select natural supplements to support and sustain these processes, etc.). Remember, an excellent state of health promotes optimal healing.

Much like treating wounds with PRP, the best results for stem cell therapy in wounds are achieved after careful and knowledgeable debridement and preparation of the wound to reduce bio-burden, devitalized tissue, and infectious material. Stem cells are mixed with PRP and placed or injected directly into and around the wound bed, and some stem cells are usually administered intravenously (IV).

Stem cells given by IV are very anti-inflammatory and have a whole-body healing effect. Infusion of stem cells is especially successful in conjunction with preparing your body (as outlined in the preceding chapters) and preparing your wound bed. Wound debridement first provides the acute injury state which causes on-site cells to release specific biochemical signals which help tell the stem cells how they need to differentiate to help augment, replace, or repair the diseased or distressed tissue.

AUTOLOGOUS STEM CELL THERAPY

Autologous stem cell therapy is a fantastic way to jump-start or move the healing process along in challenging and difficult to heal wounds. In this process, cells are taken directly from a patient's own body. The two most common methods of harvesting mesenchymal stem cells (MSCs—the ones that differentiate into skin, soft tissue, and connective tissue needed for healing wounds) are to either take them from adipose tissue (fat) or bone marrow.

Adipose tissue harvest requires a minor liposuction procedure to remove some fat from a patient's flanks or abdomen. The procedure is done under local anesthesia and typically only slightly uncomfortable. A small (approximately one-half centimeter) incision is made and subcutaneous fat is sucked out with a special suction catheter.

Alternatively, bone marrow can be removed, usually from the pelvic bone just above the buttocks, with a large needle under local anesthesia.

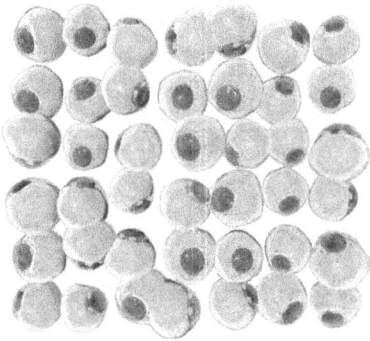

Fat cells aspirated from human adipose tissue (adipocytes)

Once the fat or bone marrow is harvested, stem cells can be isolated from the sample, typically in a few hours. Special cell counters allow us to know how many cells have been harvested and usually literally thirty million to several hundred million nucleated stem cells are obtained. There are many ways to administer stem cells, and there are currently active, ongoing, experimental studies for a variety of medical indications.

To date, the most successful published results for autologous stem cell therapy have been in orthopedic conditions such as arthritic knees, hips, and shoulders. Significant success has also been achieved with stem cell therapy in treating chronic obstructive pulmonary disease, generalized muscular decline, ischemic heart disease, and even some neurodegenerative diseases such as Parkinson's disease, multiple sclerosis, strokes, and in some cases there have been positive results with Alzheimer's disease. Obviously, the exact type of cells and the delivery method is crucial. In addition, the way the cells are separated from the fat or bone marrow is also very important, and it is critical that a validated, well-studied process is used that maximizes both cell yield and viability.

As you might expect, there are several publications showing autologous stem cell therapy to be extremely effective in treating chronic wounds. It is the next step up from using platelet rich plasma therapy. PRP delivers important and necessary growth factors to the wound and stimulates the stem cells that are already there to proliferate, differentiate, and help heal and fill in the wound. Stem cell therapy adds in a source of cells that have not previously been in the wound. These additional cells, when stimulated by the local wound environment, can multiply and differentiate into skin, connective tissue, cartilage, and whatever other tissues the body needs in that location to close the wound.

It is truly an amazing way to tap the body's own healing capacity. It is like putting an intelligent, living bandage—created by your body—onto your wound.

CORD BLOOD CELLULAR ALLOGRAFTS

For some patients, there may be an alternative, potentially more effective, and less invasive way to harness the potential of stem cells. In 2004, scientists were surprised to find that damaged organs were repairing themselves in children who had received cord blood transfusions. Stem cells had apparently traveled in their blood to other areas of the body and had grown new tissues (organs, muscle, and skin). Umbilical cord blood can be harvested from otherwise discarded umbilical cords from natural full-term births of donor mothers screened for known infections and other diseases.

There are some companies creating "cellular allografts" from healthy umbilical cords following a normal delivery. Umbilical cord stem cells have special markers on their surface, which render them immunologically privileged—the immune system of the person receiving them is programmed to ignore them and not cause rejection reactions. Usually the cells are carefully frozen (cryopreserved) using methods developed to maximize viability and then thawed before administration.

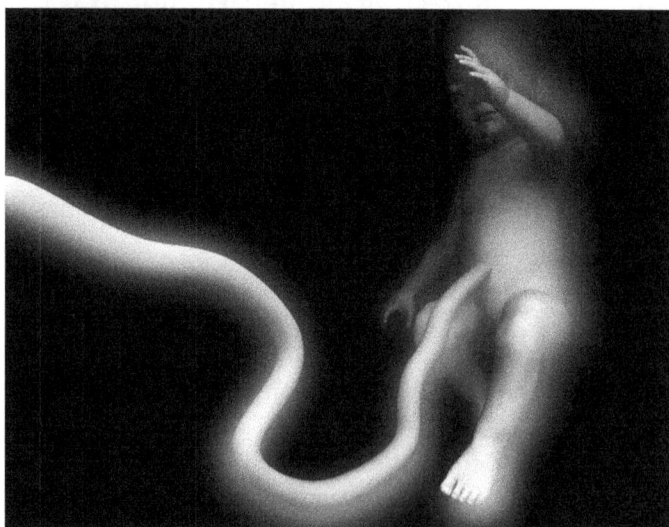

Because the mesenchymal and hematopoietic stem cells in these samples are only nine months old when they are harvested, they may have even greater ability to differentiate and regenerate tissue than stem cells derived from adult tissues. There is some debate as to whether thawed samples contain living cells or just extremely potent growth factors and other beneficial cytokines. Whether or not it is the growth factors or the cells, the effects can be impressive.

Why might you want to receive one of these cellular allografts rather than your own cells? As you age, your own stem cell supply can be compromised by age itself, major illness, injury, or toxins such as heavy metals, inflammatory conditions, etc. You might be a good candidate for an allograft product rather than autologous stem cells if you have or have had cancer, are extremely thin, have diabetes, smoke, are over the age of sixty, have autoimmune disease, or are generally unhealthy.

THE "WILD WEST" AND THE REGULATORY ENVIRONMENT

Stem cell therapy has tremendous promise in changing medicine and improving the lives of millions. The public senses that, and it has created an environment ripe for the exploitation of that hope for therapy for many challenging conditions. This has allowed many unscrupulous practitioners to charge exorbitant prices for therapies of questionable and not necessarily proven efficacy. There has been a proliferation of practitioners advertising "stem cell therapy" that ranges from simply giving PRP, to off label use of cellular allografts, to using autologous adipose or bone marrow harvested stem cells processed by any number of methods which have not necessarily been shown to effectively isolate viable stem cells.

There are, of course, many excellent practitioners who use validated techniques to isolate and administer autologous stem cell, and there are several research projects taking place both in academia and the private sector working toward developing marketable allogeneic stem cell products for many different disease states. As you can imagine, it takes hundreds of millions of dollars to develop a product like this, prove its safety, prove its efficacy for a disease process, and bring it to market. That, coupled with the public controversy about embryonic stem cells as we mentioned (which has sometimes made funding for research difficult to come by), has made bringing viable products to market very slow.

Currently, there are countries where one can go to get various types of stem cell therapy where the regulatory scrutiny is considerably less (for example, several Caribbean Islands have made very favorable laws regarding the administration of stem cells, including "culture expanded" cells). But, as they say, "Buyer, beware!" You may not always be getting what you think; you certainly hope it is safe and effective for the condition you are seeking treatment for.

In the United States, the Food and Drug Administration (FDA) is currently looking at how to regulate stem cell therapy to make sure that patients get safe and effective treatments. Although the FDA has traditionally had regulatory power over pharmaceuticals (drugs) and medical devices, it also has regulatory power over biologic and tissue products, and it is under that rubric that stem cell therapy will ultimately be viewed. The counter argument by many physicians has been that stem cell therapy is more like a surgical procedure such as a skin graft—taking a piece of tissue and moving it from one place to another—and that is not something the FDA is able to regulate. Nonetheless, the FDA is moving to regulate stem cell therapy under the precept that the tissue that the cells are coming from is more than "minimally manipulated" and that the cells are not necessarily for "homologous use."

For now, our recommendations are as follows: It is important to ask any doctor delivering stem cell therapy about their training and credentials. Look for doctors who are fellowship-trained, familiar with the regulatory environment surrounding SCT, work under approved experimental protocols, are affiliated with an institutional review board (IRB), and are looking to improve, publish, and report their outcomes to the public. Make sure you understand what the source of the cells is, how they are being processed, and what data they have on efficacy, in addition to what their experience and training is. Our hope is that a few years from now SCT will have proven itself and no longer be considered experimental, so that the promise of these amazing techniques becomes easier for patients to access and can be helpful to many more patients.

We expect many changes in the field over the next few years, and we will stay abreast with them to be able to continue to deliver only the highest quality and most efficacious stem cell therapy to our patients. We believe these therapies can improve the lives of millions, perhaps billions of people with wounds from around the world.

References and Recommended Reading

1. Smith, Robin L. *Healing Cell: How the Greatest Revolution in Medical History Is Changing Your Life*. Center St, 2014. Print.

2. Furcht, Leo. *Stem Cell Dilemma: Beacons of Hope or Harbingers of Doom?* W W Norton, 2011. Print.

3. Steenblock D, and Payne A. *Umbilical Cord Stem Cell Therapy, The Gift of Healing from Healthy Newborns*. Basic Health Publications, 2006. Print.

4. Dougherty EJ. "An evidence-based model comparing the cost-effectiveness of platelet-rich plasma gel to alternative therapies for patients with non-healing diabetic foot ulcers." *Adv Skin Wound Care*. 2008; 21(12), 568-75.

5. Lacci KM, Dardik A. "Platelet Rich Plasma: Support for Its Use in Wound Healing." *Yale J Biology & Med. 2010; 83(210): 1-9*

6. Hanson SE, et al. "Mesenchymal Stem Cell Therapy for Non-healing Cutaneous Wounds." *Plast Reconstr Surg. 2010; 125(2): 510-516.*

7. Wu Y, et al. "Mesenchymal Stem Cells Enhance Wound Healing Through Differentiation and Angiogenesis." *Stem Cells*. 2007; 25(10): 2548-2659.

8. Menendez-Menendez Y, Alvarez-Viejo M, Ferrero-Gutierrez A, Perez-Basterrechea M, Perez Lopez S et al. (2014) "Adult Stem Cell

WOUND HEALING SECRETS

Therapy in Chronic Wound Healing." *J Stem Cell Res Ther* 4:162. doi:10.4172/2157-7633.1000162

9. Huang SP, et al. "Promotion of wound healing using adipose derived stem cells in radiation ulcer of a rat model." *J Biomed Science.* 2013; 20:51.

10. Millman JR, Xie C, van Dervort A, Gürtler M, Pagliuca FW, Melton DA. "Generation of stem cell-derived ß cells from patients with type 1 diabetes." *Nature Communications.* May 10, 2016. DOI: 10.1038/ncomms11463

CHAPTER 20

Introducing the Quantlet

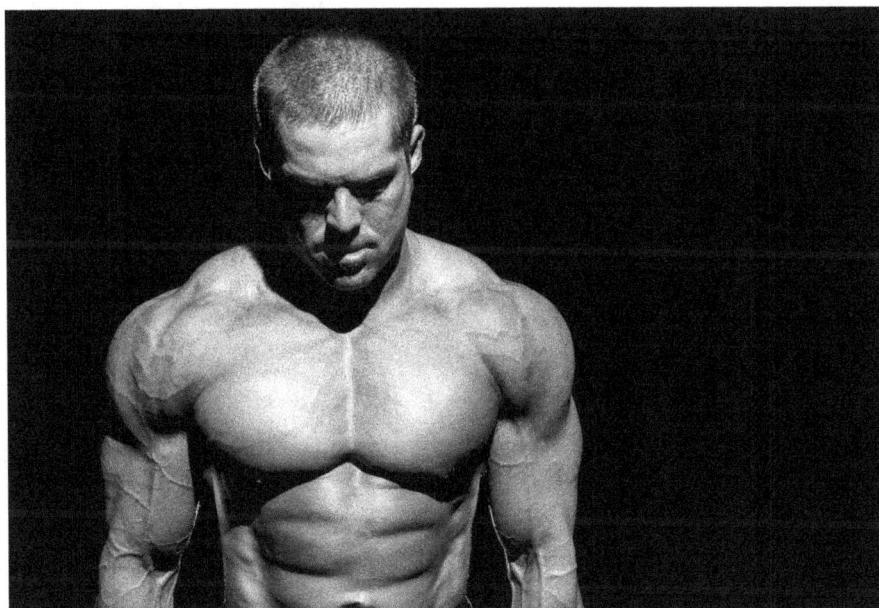

We want to take the opportunity to introduce you to a device which is not yet available at the time of this writing, but one that we sincerely believe will have significant effects on wound healing based on its operating principles. We are acquainted with the developers of this device, the technology that it uses, and some of the early data and testing. It relies heavily on the emerging understanding of quantum biology and mitochondrial energetics, both of which are critical to wound healing. It is portable, battery-powered, and may be used on any limb. Although it will have a significant systemic effect if worn on the wrist as designed, the capability of moving it to a problematic area closer to or even on a wound will be significant. We anticipate that using it on the legs, either directly on the wound or on the arterial circulation there, will have a significant local effect that will positively impact healing.

Although the device is a consumer grade device and not specifically intended, labeled, or studied for medical uses, early results have suggested to us that it may have significant positive health benefits, particularly in those with the chronic conditions that cause wounds (diabetes, peripheral vascular disease, autoimmune disease, venous insufficiency, and inflammatory conditions). It has been designed primarily for augmenting human athletic performance, improving sleep, and promoting general health and wellness. We cannot wait to use it on our wound patients, as we believe it will have a tremendous effect on not only healing their wounds but improving general health.

The device of which we speak is called "The Quantlet." More information can be found at www.TheQuantlet.com.

WHAT DOES IT DO?

The Quantlet specifically does two things:

- It cools the body and thus the bloodstream. It has a thermoelectric cooler unit which helps slightly lower body temperature, not enough to make you cold or hypothermic but enough to make a difference in cellular energetics.

- It delivers several different frequencies of light, specifically in frequencies centered around red and purple, to the bloodstream.

You may be wondering how that helps heal your wounds.

WHY DOES COOLING HELP?

Cooling the bloodstream (and the rest of the body) is a technique that works on the physical properties of materials. You may recall from physics and chemistry that when a substance is heated, the atoms and molecules vibrate more and tend to be farther apart. Cooling causes the converse; it removes thermal energy from the system, decreases the vibration of molecules, and consequently allows them to be closer together.

The distance between molecules, particularly in the mitochondria, is critical to how quickly the important bio-chemical and biophysical reactions that create ATP, the body's energy currency, can take place. Just moving some of the critical enzymes of the electron chain transport (ECT) proteins one angstrom (10-10 meters—or 0.000000001 meter) closer together can increase the electron tunneling potential by a factor of ten. This has a huge impact on your body's ability to produce the critical energy needed for wound healing.

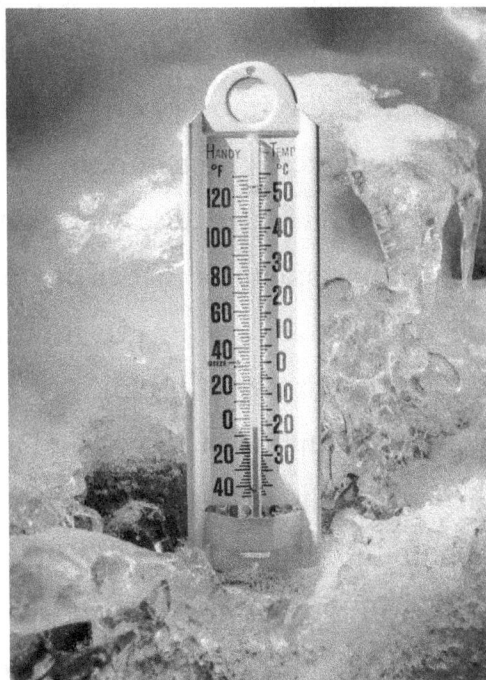

We are not going to go into the details of quantum physics which this describes, but suffice it to say that the easier it is for electrons to tunnel and create reactions in the ECT, the more energy your body can produce, the better and faster you heal. Healing your wound takes a lot of energy, and the chronic diseases that cause the wounds that you have are usually the result of (and/or the cause of) significantly disordered mitochondrial energetics. Thus, increasing the ability of your mitochondria to produce energy will vastly improve your ability to heal.

Much of this is based on some new information about the cause of disease in human beings. The mainstream and traditional medical approach to human disease has been to look for dysfunction at the organ system, organ, or cellular level. New techniques and emerging science are teaching us that many diseases that we cannot explain using this perspective are likely caused by dysfunction of the mitochondria within an organ system. For example, dementia, cognitive decline, and mental illness are related to the inability of the mitochondrial in the neurologic system (brain) to produce the requisite energy to keep the neurologic system working correctly. Likewise, heart failure is ultimately produced by failure of the mitochondria within the heart muscle. Mitochondrial dysfunction, or inefficient function, in any system of the body will lead to disorder, chaos, and ultimately disease in that system.

The bottom line is that an organism without energy is dead, and so increasing an organism's energy gets it farther from death, which is a somewhat odd but apt description of health.

The technique of using the blood vessels of the hand and wrist to cool the body has been tested extensively at Stanford University. Researchers there have found that cooling takes advantage of the arterial-venous anastomoses (AVAs) in the palm of the hand, is an effective way of slightly lowering body temperature, and creates incredible improvements in athletic performance. (For example, one subject went from being able to do 180 pull-ups to 620 pull-ups over a six-week period!) Although your goal may not be to improve your athletic performance, the same techniques that increase the ability of athletes to perform will increase the ability of your body to heal your wounds.

WHAT ABOUT LIGHT?

The other action of the Quantlet is to "infuse" light into the bloodstream. This is done by precisely placing light-emitting diodes (LEDs) over the radial and ulnar arteries of the wrist. As we have talked about previously in the book, light has a tremendous effect on human biology, and using the right frequencies of light, combined with cold to improve electron flow, will be a game-changer. There has been a tremendous amount of research on light and the technique of photobiomodulation—using light to influence biologic function—which is just starting to come into focus in terms of therapeutic value. As we have discussed, some of the advanced therapies used to treat wounds include specific light therapies (THOR Laser, Delta Laser, UV/red lights).

What does light do? Light is energy, and the amount of energy that any individual photon (the tiniest "unit" or "particle" of light) carries is expressed by the "color" of the light. At one end of the spectrum, with the highest energy, is ultraviolet (UV) light, which starts with frequencies just higher than purple light and extends quickly into not being visible. UV has a very high frequency and a short wavelength and, at the wrong time and in the wrong tissues, UV light can damage tissue. However, the high energy of UV light is critical to building exclusion zones (EZs) in intracellular water, and the energy that UV light carries, when properly transduced by certain molecules in the body (such as hemoglobin and DHA), helps add to whole body energetics.

For more on exclusion zones and what is known as the "fourth phase of water," we would refer you to Dr. Gerald Pollack's excellent book of that name, as referenced in the additional reading section.

Although the relevance of this to biology is just starting to be realized, it appears that intracellular EZs in water may be one of the primary quantum mechanisms by which our cells are energized and our bodies are powered. Remember, a body without energy is a corpse, and the bio-energetic perspective of human health postulates that your state of health is directly proportional to the amount of energy that your body carries, produces, and can process.

If you wonder whether UV light really has any kind of biologic relevance, then you should know that the human hemoglobin molecule has the same structure as the chlorophyll molecule in plants, with the only difference being that hemoglobin has an iron atom in the center, and chlorophyll has a magnesium atom in the center. The structure of both molecules is otherwise the same, and it is exquisitely tuned to respond to light in the UV frequency range.

At the other end of the spectrum from UV is red light, which has a relatively lower frequency and longer wavelength than UV, and does not carry nearly as much energy. Beyond the visible red light of the spectrum is infrared, which we perceive as heat. Red and infrared light, both of which are used in the Quantlet, have frequencies which have been found to have numerous biologic benefits including improving circulation, stimulating angiogenesis (the formation of new blood vessels), promoting phagocytosis (the process of immune system cells engulfing (gobbling up) foreign material and organisms), increasing lymphatic activity, stimulating fibroblast production, increasing collagen production, and promoting tissue granulation.

Two other critical actions of red light that may be at the root of the others listed are the fact that it is known to enhance the activity of an enzyme called cytochrome c oxidase. This enzyme is part of the critical steps of the electron chain transport in mitochondria, which produce ATP, the cellular energy currency that we all need to carry out every function in our body. The more ATP your body can make, the more energy it has available.

Finally, at the subatomic (quantum) level, it appears that it is infrared light (lower in frequency and longer in wavelength than even red light) that creates exclusion zones in intracellular water. So EZ water in your cells, which acts like an atomic scale battery that stores energy, is created initially by the action of infrared light on cells, and the EZ is made larger by light in the purple and UV part of the frequency range—i.e., more energy can be stored in it. In summary, the right frequencies of light, some of which will be used in the Quantlet, create and store more energy in your body's batteries, while the cooling provided increases the efficiency and energy production of those batteries.

SUMMARY

Although the Quantlet is not yet available to the general public at the time of this writing, it is currently in beta-testing (anticipated release fourth quarter of 2017), it combines two critically important modalities that independently improve human bioenergetics and health. Non-healing wound patients are

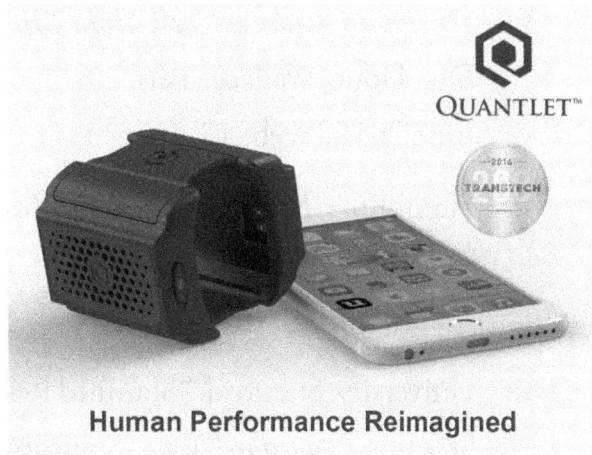

Human Performance Reimagined

always very deficient in intracellular energy, and both cold thermogenesis and light therapy have been shown to have significant impacts on healing wounds through a variety of physiologic mechanisms, some of the very basics of which are detailed here.

As physicians, we believe that the synergistic combination of these two modalities, combined into one easily portable, rechargeable, reasonably priced, consumer grade device will be a tremendous boon to all who suffer from chronic wounds. If you are interested in more information, please go to the website (www.theQuantlet.com) or see the additional information on our website (www.quantumhealthandhealing.com). We expect continued refinements of this and similar devices using the dual modalities it employs will be hugely beneficial to healing.

References and Recommended Reading

1. Pollack, Gerald H. *The Fourth Phase of Water: Beyond Solid, Liquid, and Vapor*. Seattle: Ebner & Sons, 2013. Print.

2. Kruse, Jack, MD. "Cold Thermogenesis Easy Start Guide." *Living an Optimized Life*. Www.jackkruse.com, Web. 12 Apr. 2017.

3. *Dr. Doug Wallace - Talk from 8th Annual Oliver Smithies Symposium*. Dir. Doug Wallace. Perf. Dr. Doug Wallace. *YouTube*. YouTube, 16 June 2015. Web. 12 Apr. 2017.

4. Hamblin, Michael, PhD. "Mechanisms of Low Level Light Therapy." *MECHANISMS OF LOW LEVEL LIGHT THERAPY*. Web. 12 Apr. 2017.

5. University, Stanford. "Stanford Researchers' Cooling Glove 'better than Steroids'." *Stanford News*. Stanford University, 29 Aug. 2012. Web. 12 Apr. 2017."The Quantlet® – Human Performance Reimagined." *The Quantlet by Quantum Dynamics LLC*. Web. 12 Apr. 2017.

6. Quantum Dynamics LLC. "The Quantlet - Human Performance Reimagined." The Quantlet. Web12 April 2017.

CHAPTER 21

Next Steps: Your Pathway to Healing

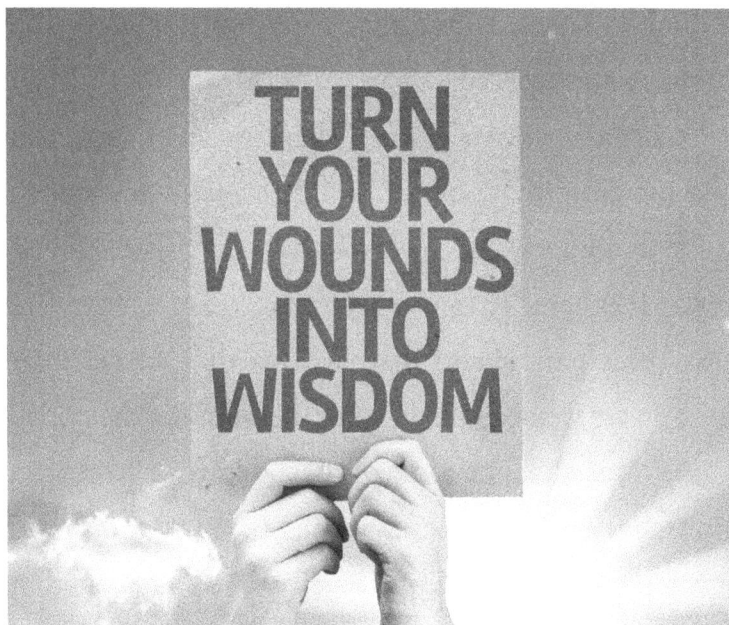

Our combined expertise and study of quantum biology allows us to evaluate non-healing wounds from a different perspective. As you have heard, quantum health and healing means using nature and biology to heal. If you heal your body, it becomes much more likely that you will heal your wound (and avoid cancer, diabetes, heart disease, etc.). Heal your body, and then watch your wound heal as a result.

We have blended our conventional medical backgrounds and expertise while adding our alternative and regenerative medicine knowledge. For your wound to really progress, you need the best of both medical "worlds." The traditional medical "gold standard" is often unreliable, too lengthy, very costly, and sometimes difficult to access given the jumbled and fragmented healthcare system. We utilize a holistic approach and natural methods to heal the patients we treat. In addition, we always create a personalized wound treatment plan.

Too often, a non-healing wound, which is most often seen in people beyond fifty years of age, is accepted as an aging problem. It is actually a lifestyle problem. Poor sleep habits, lack of regular, sensible exercise, poor nutrition and dietary habits, high levels of daily stress, EMF, and toxins in air and water all work against a proper oxygen supply to our organs and tissues, and the result is chronic disease and chronic wounds. If there are any methods of influencing or correcting for the daily abuse of our bodies, and maintaining and increasing our quality of life at all ages, and reversing a diverse spectrum of diseases and ailments, why not try them?

The more we study natural and alternative medicine based on the physics of biology, the more aware we become of issues that prevent the body from healing. We hope you have learned about some of these and ways to correct them.

Our environment is not the same as our parents' and grandparents'. We live in an environment of increasing toxicity. We told you that one way to detoxify your body is to drink a lot of good quality water. This helps your body release toxins through the kidneys, sweating, tears, and bowel movements. We recommend a reverse osmosis water-filtering unit or drinking fresh spring water. Tap water has become increasingly contaminated.

The worse your diet, the more toxins you need to excrete (an infrared sauna can be very helpful here). Eating organically and avoiding GMOs helps too. We encourage a diet high in seafood (epi-paleo). We strongly recommend time outside in the sunshine whenever possible. Naturally synthesized vitamin D is best, and the sun also provides light energy to our cells' mitochondria.

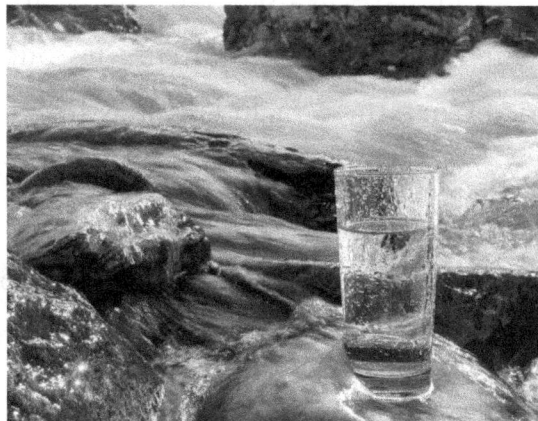

Another critical part of optimal health and healing is paying attention to circadian cycles. Turn off the lights not long after sundown and wear blue-light blocking eyewear, go to bed earlier, and avoid artificial sources of light after dark. These include your TV, computer screens, Kindles, iPads, and smart-phones. Sleep is critical for the healing and restoration of your body. You will find that your biologic rhythms adjust, and this takes you a long way toward better health and healing.

Hopefully, a better understanding of quantum biology has revealed how you can stimulate your body's own regenerative processes to heal *your* wound. We are committed to researching and keeping up with the latest in medical and scientific innovations in tissue repair and healing to improve our patients' outcomes (for example, the Quantlet device). We continue to research new ideas, such as nitrous oxide and peptide therapies. You deserve *healing* AND *health* restoration.

We have discussed many things in this book, from significant lifestyle changes, to causative factors for wounds, to specific topical treatments for wounds and how to take care of them at home, to medical treatment such as bio-identical hormone replacement. You have learned how earthing, nutrition, and supplements can improve cellular metabolism and promote healing.

You have heard about some advanced therapies that will help heal your wounds that are oftentimes outside the tunnel vision of mainstream medicine. These include things like stem cell therapy, platelet rich plasma, advanced wound dressings, ozone therapy, microcurrent, light/laser therapy, and others.

You may be wondering what to do next. This has been a lot of information and, unfortunately, we have had to focus on breadth rather than depth. Nearly any one of the things we have talked about in this book could literally be a chapter or potentially even a book unto itself. We look forward to helping disseminate more information to you in the future.

Properly healing your wound requires a balanced combination of these methods. If you have a chronic wound, and we have said it many times, you have not attained the state of health that will help you heal. Diligent attention to many of the lifestyle modifications mentioned in the book will help improve your general state of health and significantly increase your chance of healing—and rate of healing.

Beyond that, it will be important to partner with a physician or other practitioner who understands the nuances of healing chronic wounds and which therapies are most likely to help at which point of the wound-healing process. People with any type of chronic medical problem struggle to find the best doctor, the best treatments, and the best way to make life easier and pain-free. It should be no different with a chronic wound. Their expertise has usually been gained through hard experience and seeing thousands of wounds. We cannot recommend enough that you seek out a local qualified practitioner, usually best found at a specialty wound care center (because it is a relatively new specialty, request the most experienced physician).

It would also behoove you to find and partner with a physician trained in functional and integrative medicine who can help you manage your hormones and who may offer you some of the advanced and alternative therapies described in this book. Someone who will help you reverse disease (naturally), not treat the *symptoms* of disease (with pharmaceuticals).

We have just scratched the surface here on how to help you heal. But we hope in doing so, that we have been able to give you hope that there is a way to heal every chronic wound. There is no reason that you should have to suffer with a non-healing wound. You need not end up with an amputation.

We are not saying healing is necessarily easy, and it certainly will not happen without your active involvement and hard work (usually meaning significant lifestyle changes) and qualified practitioners. The techniques in this book have made a positive difference in the lives of so many people with wounds. We hope it will be of value to you too.

We realize that this book does not tell you all the information you need. We could not describe all of our modalities in the book, but if you are interested, we would be happy to send you free reports. If you would like to regularly receive more information and new updates on ways to heal your wound, just visit our websites, www.woundhealingsecrets.com and www.healingyourwound.com, and sign up for our email list and ask us questions. We would love to continue to help you understand how quantum healing not only helps improve your wound but also is able to eliminate some of the worst diseases of our time.

At our clinic, we focus on wellness. We spend most our time educating our patients so that they can better understand their medical conditions. In the words of Dr. Jack Kruse, "When it becomes easier to prescribe than to educate, the doctor has lost his or her edge." Knowledge empowers you to become well and stay in charge of your health. Who knows? Maybe your wound will be your "wake up call" to better health. It is better than "waking up" once you have suffered an amputation.

To better health and healing,
Drs. Julie and Rob Hamilton

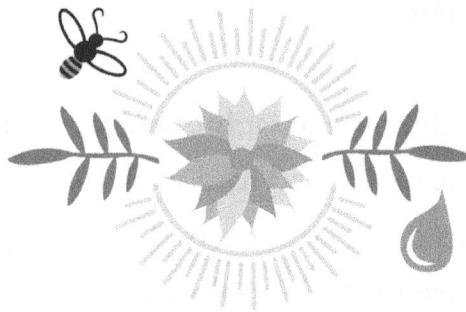

WOUND
HEALING SECRETS
SAVING LIFE AND LIMB